Interferons
A PRIMER

Interferons

A PRIMER

ROBERT M. FRIEDMAN

Laboratory of Experimental Pathology
National Institute of Arthritis,
Metabolism, and Digestive Diseases
National Institutes of Health
Bethesda, Maryland

1981

ACADEMIC PRESS

A Subsidiary of Harcourt Brace Jovanovich, Publishers

New York   London   Toronto   Sydney   San Francisco

ACADEMIC PRESS, INC.
111 Fifth Avenue, New York, New York 10003

United Kingdom Edition published by
ACADEMIC PRESS, INC. (LONDON) LTD.
24/28 Oval Road, London NW1 7DX

Library of Congress Cataloging in Publication Data

Friedman, Robert M.
    Interferons: a primer.

    Includes bibliographies and index.
    1. Interferon.   I. Title. [DNLM: 1. Interferon.
QW 800 F862i]
QR187.5.F74   616.07'9   81-2887
ISBN 0-12-268280-7   AACR2

PRINTED IN THE UNITED STATES OF AMERICA

81 82 83 84   9 8 7 6 5 4 3 2 1

CONTENTS

v

PREFACE

So many specialized books are published in the biological sciences that it has become the custom for an author to defend his or her writing the work in question. Therefore, like other authors, I feel I must say something at the start about the origin and purpose of this book.

Because there have been several excellent advanced books recently published on the details of the interferon system, there is presently no need for yet another text on interferons. However, these texts are difficult to use if one is *not* an expert. Since there is no volume available for the student, scientist, physician, or educated layperson who wishes to know something about interferons, but who is not planning to carry out research in this area, I resolved to write such a book. This primer is the result of that effort.

I have been doing research on interferons since 1960, when I came to work with Dr. Sam Baron at NIH to investigate why animals recovered from primary virus infections. We became aware of Isaacs' discovery of interferons at that time and concluded that they might well contribute to recovery from some primary virus infections.

After a residency in pathology at the Clinical Center of the NIH, during which I worked with Dr. Alan Rabson on the possible role of interferons in determining the oncogenic potential of variants of polyoma virus, I spent a year in Alick Isaacs' laboratory at Mill Hill, which at that time was the place to go for interferon research. Most of the important work in the field was then being carried out by Isaacs. Unfortunately, I was only able to work with Isaacs for four months before the tragic illness began that two years later was to claim his life. Because of Isaacs' absence most of that year, the postdoctoral fellows in the laboratory, Joseph Sonnabend, Joyce Taylor-Papadrimitriou, and I plodded on alone with work on the biochemistry mechanism of interferon action.

I returned to the Laboratory of Pathology of the National Cancer Institute in late 1964 to continue my work on the mechanism of interferon's antiviral activity. Between 1964 and 1971, I worked under Drs. Harold Stewart and Louis Thomas on several aspects of interferon production, action, and antiviral activity in animals together with Sam Baron, Hilton Levy, and Phil Grimley, among others. In 1971 I returned to Mill Hill for two years to work with Ian Kerr on the effect of interferon on virus protein synthesis in cell-free systems. After this exciting experience I returned to the NIH, but this time to the Laboratory of Experimental Pathology in the Arthritis Institute (NIAMDD). Since that time I have had the pleasure of working with many other researchers at NIH and elsewhere.

In retrospect, I was first attracted to the study of interferons because of the selective nature of their potentially useful biological effect. Because interferons seemed to inhibit the replication processes of viruses and not to inhibit cells, they seemed like natural antivirals with possible therapeutic applications. Therefore, it has been of great interest to me to watch the explosive expansion of this field in recent years. It now seems that interferons do many things besides inhibiting virus replication. They seem to modulate cell growth and regulate some aspects of the immune system. What a surprise to find so many applications for something you have been familiar with for twenty years!

I often wonder what Alick Isaacs would have thought of the developments in "his" area of research. He would, of course, have been delighted with the vast range of biological applications of his discovery. At the same time, his puckish humor would have enabled him to find irony in the fact that it was his original description of interferon as an antiviral substance that effectively put blinders on almost everyone who subsequently worked with interferons. When we came across what were non-antiviral actions of interferon, we dismissed them as due to contaminants in the preparations. How wrong we all were! Perhaps if Isaacs had lived longer, his intuition would have set us right sooner.

Intuition is the right word to use in the case of Alick Isaacs. The discovery with Jean Lindermann in 1957 of interferon was just one, although the most remarkable, of the achievements of Isaac's career. There were many clues in the work of many scientists carried on before 1957 that could well have led to the discovery of the nonspecific, antiviral substances that we now call interferons. Even going back to Jenner's studies on cowpox and smallpox, such a resistance factor may have been recognized. It was Isaacs, though, who made the logical jump to the notion that the nonspecific resistance factor was humoral. At first, this insight was so revolutionary that the very existence of interferon was doubted in the best circles in virology. It was, in fact, dubbed "imaginon" by some scientists who now spend a great deal of their time working on interferons. However, the magnitude of Isaacs' contribution is now quite evident.

Although I have been involved with interferons for a long time, I am still very excited by their biological and their medical potential. One purpose of this book is to share some of my excitement with others who I consider only in this case less fortunate than I am. I hope this book does transmit some of my sense of excitement to the nonspecialists in interferon for whom it was intended. I have included a glossary at the end of the book for those to whom the terminology used may be unfamiliar; I trust this section will allow the book to be read and understood by a larger group than would have otherwise been possible.

A few thanks are in order. First, I would like to thank my

family for the many years of patience they have shown during the development and fruition, such as it is, of my career in interferon research. Next, I would like to thank the men who taught me virology: Mark Adams, Alick Isaacs, Alan Rabson, and Sam Baron. The first two died at such a young age that it is painful to think of them and all they could have accomplished. Sam and Al fortunately go on and are so wholesome they are likely to continue forever. I sincerely hope so.

I would also like to give my thanks to Hilton Levy, George Galasso, and especially to T. Sreevalsan, who have critically read this manuscript. Finally, many thanks to my secretary, Ms. Joan Mok. There is no way this book could have been started or finished without her help.

Robert M. Friedman

1
INTRODUCTION

Viruses are intracellular parasites that are smaller than bacteria. Their structure contains a ribonucleic or deoxyribonucleic acid, one or more proteins, and in some cases lipids. Viral proteins may be functional enzymes, but most viruses depend on cellular enzymes to carry out the synthetic processes necessary for their growth. Viruses attach to cells and enter them. Their nucleic acid then subverts the normal growth and maintenance processes of the cell and converts the cell into a factory for producing viruses.

In order to inhibit virus growth selectively, it is necessary to find substances that are toxic to the virus, but that do not harm the cell. Because of the intimate association of virus growth with the normal cellular metabolic machinery, this is not an easy task. Antibiotics and other antimicrobials are effective on bacteria, fungi, or parasites because the metabolism of these infectious agents is often so different from that of the cell that it has not been difficult to find agents selectively toxic for them; not so with viruses. Only recently has some progress been made in finding effective antiviral drugs.

What is an effective antiviral drug for humans? Primarily it must inhibit virus growth at concentrations that are relatively nontoxic to human cells. It must be active in all types of cells. To make the antiviral drug particularly useful, it should also possess a wide spectrum of antiviral activity, so that the growth of most human disease-causing viruses will be inhibited following treatment with it. In many ways, interferons are ideal antiviral substances.

2

Interferons are proteins that exert a wide-spectrum antiviral activity in animal cells and also possess several biological activities other than the ability to induce an antiviral state. An interferon is often active only in cells of the animal species producing that interferon; cellular metabolic processes involving both RNA and protein synthesis are required for development of interferon activity. Concentrations of interferons that induce significant levels of biological activity usually cause little or no toxic effect on cells. Interferon production is induced by viruses or a number of antiviral substances.

Interferons were discovered in the late 1950s by Isaacs and Lindenmann, who were working then at Mill Hill in London. They were at the time investigating a phenomenon called viral interference. Viral interference can be defined simply as the ability of one virus to interfere with the growth of another virus. The viruses may be similar or entirely unrelated. No mechanism of action is specified by the term *interference*, but now we know several mechanisms that may be involved (Table I). For instance, infected cells may produce virus particles that are called defective interfering particles (DIPs); these inhibit the synthesis of complete virus nucleic acids. Also, some viruses inhibit the absorption of other viruses by blocking their sites of attachment.

It is characteristic of most (the exception being intrinsic interference) instances of noninterferon, viral interference that the inhibition is between closely related viruses, is rapid in onset, and can be reversed by washing. These properties are in contrast to the mechanism of interferon action discussed below. One paradox should be mentioned to avoid later confusion: the various antiviral mechanisms of interferon action appear to involve at least two of those steps listed in Table I. Although the actual actions of in-

TABLE I. Types of Viral Interference That Do Not Involve Interferon

Competition for or destruction of cell receptors for viruses
Inhibition of virus penetration
Inhibition of synthesis of viral components
Inhibition of viral assembly
Intrinsic interference (applies to Newcastle disease virus only)

terferons are quite different from those of noninterferon interference, the steps of viral synthesis and virus assembly have been reported to be inhibited in interferon-treated cells.

Isaacs was working on interference with influenza virus growth when it occurred to him that perhaps it was not only the viral particle that could cause interference, but also some humoral factor or hormonelike substance that might be responsible. He therefore carried out a simple experiment; he treated membranes from chick eggs with inactivated influenza virus. The usual experiment carried out up to that time was to leave the inactivated or live virus on cells and to study the inhibition in these cells of the growth of a second virus. The unusual thing that Isaacs and Lindenmann did was to treat with the inactivated virus, wash the membranes, let them incubate for several hours, and then remove the medium. The medium was then used to treat fresh membranes that had never been exposed to virus. These latter membranes, after incubation with the fluids, were then infected with additional virus. They found that a humoral factor had indeed been produced and that factor transferred the interference. They called the factor interferon.

The basic properties of interferons were rapidly discovered by Isaacs and his co-workers at Mill Hill. The general properties of interferons are compared to antibodies in Table II.

TABLE II. Properties of Interferon and Antibody

Property	Interferon	Antibody
Glycoprotein	Often	Yes
Antiviral	Yes	Yes
Acts directly on virus particles	No	Yes
Virus specific in action	No	Yes
Acts through cells	Yes	No
Cell species specificity	Often	Never
Produced in specialized cells	No[a]	Yes
Induced by antigen	On reexposure only	Yes

[a] Gamma interferon is an exception to this rule.

Both antibodies and interferons are antiviral, but, although interferons do not act directly on intact viruses, they act directly on the cells by inducing an antiviral state. The development of antiviral activity requires metabolic activity on the part of the cells. If cellular RNA or protein synthesis is inhibited, so is the development of the antiviral state. The antiviral state induced by interferons is directed against a wide variety of viruses, in marked contrast to the specificity of antibodies that can distinguish between subtypes of viruses.

Many interferons tend to be species specific in action, an unusual but not unique biological property. For instance, chick interferon is completely inactive on human cells; however, human alpha interferon is active not only on human cells but on pig, cow, and the cells of several other varieties of animal, so that the species specificity of interferon is not absolute.

One interesting similarity between interferons and antibodies is that antibodies and one type of interferon (immune or gamma interferon) are both produced in response to a specific antigen. Antibodies are produced on first exposure of an immunocyte to an antigen; interferons, on the other hand, require previous sensitization. However, antibodies are produced only by cells of the immune system, whereas different interferons may be produced by cells of the immune system as well as by fibroblasts or epithelial cells. In fact, almost every cell type has been reported to produce at least one type of interferon, but the amount of interferon produced by any one cell tends to be small, possibly because of very high biological activity of interferons.

Other properties of interferons should be noted at this point. The biological activity of most interferons is remarkably stable; it survives treatment at very acid pH (indeed most interferons are stable at a pH of 2), with ionic detergents such as sodium dodecyl sulfate, or with sulfhydryl reagents such as mercaptoethanol. Most interferons also tend to be thermostable.

Figure 1 briefly summarizes the production and action of interferons. A cell is induced to make an interferon by infection with a virus or by exposure to a variety of nonviral substances that are known to be interferon inducers. In a variable time period after exposure to an interferon inducer the cell elaborates a spe-

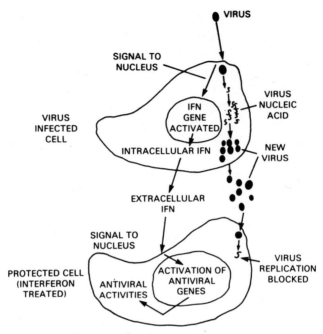

Fig. 1. Interferon production and action.

The upper cell is infected with a virus, but interferon may also be induced by nonviral substances. The virus is uncoated to yield a nucleic acid that replicates to form new viral nucleic acid and protein. New virus is assembled and released from the cell into the extracellular fluid. One or more aspects of the virus replication process are interpreted by the genetic apparatus of the cell as an activation signal for interferon production. The interferon gene is activated so that interferon is produced within the cell, and also released into the extracellular fluid. This interferon interacts with another cell, probably by binding to its surface. This binding signals the activation of the antiviral genes in the nucleus of the cell and several antiviral activities are produced. An antiviral state then exists within the cytoplasm so that the cell is protected from subsequent virus infections. When such a protected cell is infected with a virus, the virus can absorb to the cell, enter it, and uncoat normally. After this stage virus replication is inhibited, so that little or no progeny virus is released.

cific messenger RNA (IFmRNA) for an interferon. The IFmRNA is then translated and the newly formed interferon glycoprotein is transported to the extracellular fluid.

Interferons seem to interact with the surface of the cell as a first step in the induction of an intracellular antiviral state. Through a number of reactions that then take place, a series of changes in intracellular enzyme levels appears to be induced by interferon treatment. These changes in enzymes—some being induced, others inhibited—give rise to the antiviral state. The alterations in enzyme levels together with changes in the morphological constituents may also be responsible for an interferon's regulatory actions on cell growth and on the immune system.

Several excellent reviews of the interferon field are available.

BIBLIOGRAPHY

Baron, S., and Dianzani, F. (eds.) (1978). The Interferon System: A current review to 1978. *Tex. Rep. Biol. Med.* **35**, 1–573. (The latter may be purchased for $10.00 from Texas Reports, Univ. of Texas Medical Branch, Galveston, Tx 77550.)

Finter, N. B. (ed.) (1973). Interferons and Interferon Inducers. Amer. Elsevier, New York.

Stewart, W. E. II. (1979). The Interferon System. Springer-Verlag, Berlin and New York.

2

ASSAYS FOR INTERFERON

Assays for interferons have so far been based on their biological activity. Most of these have involved estimates of virus growth inhibition, either by directly measuring the decrease in yield of an infectious virus or by quantitating inhibition of the production of a virus constituent or a virus function; however, because of the many biological activities of interferons, other biological assays based on inhibition of cell growth or on regulation of the immune system are possible.

It is critical to bear in mind that this is being written at a time of rapid progress in the area of interferon research. Discovery of new and exact assay methods based on the availability of purified interferons is likely in the next few years. This would include the development of a radioimmunoassay possibly employing monoclonal antibodies to specific interferons. It is important, however, to question whether such advances in methodology will improve interferon assay results, for although the biological assays for interferons tend to be slow and inexact (a twofold variation is acceptable in them), they have one enormous virtue: because of the very great biological activity of interferons, as little as 0.5 pg of interferon may be picked up in a biological assay, less than one could reasonably expect to find in most other types of assay. This extreme sensitivity has made possible, among other things, the detection of minute amounts of interferon mRNA that would have been inconceivable with a less sensitive assay. Therefore, as is often true in science, everything new may not necessarily result in an improvement.

FACTORS AFFECTING INTERFERON ASSAYS

As outlined by Finter, the ideal interferon assay would be simple, rapid, reliable, reproducible, precise, and sensitive. Biological assays fall short of most of these criteria, but not so short that they are entirely unacceptable. At least one form of the various assays discussed below should suit every need and taste.

Even in a biological assay there is one *sine qua non* that has to be met: there must be a relationship between the concentration of interferon and the response of the cells. This is met by all the assays that will be discussed. For instance, in an assay studying reduction in virus yields there is always a range (usually between 20 and 80% inhibition) where the relationship between the log of the interferon concentration and the log of the reduction in virus yield is linear. An example of this is shown in Fig. 2, which is

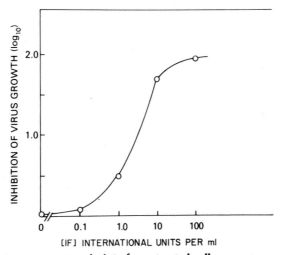

Fig. 2. Dose–response curve in interferon-treated cells.
Monolayers of primary chick embryo fibroblasts were treated for 14 hr with 0, 0.1, 1, 10, or 100 chick interferon (IF) reference units. The cells were then washed three times with medium and infected with Semliki Forest virus (SFV-arbovirus group A) at a virus-to-cell multiplicity of 20:1. After 8 hr of virus infection at the end of the rapid phase of virus replication, the cells and their medium were frozen. After thawing, the medium was assayed for yields of SFV by inhibition of plaque formation in primary chick embryo fibroblast monolayers. The virus yield with each concentration of interferon was expressed in terms of $\log_{10}$ and was subtracted from the yield of virus in the monolayer that had not been treated with interferon. This difference in virus yields was plotted as inhibition of virus growth.

taken from an experiment employing partially purified chick interferon in primary chick embryo fibroblast cultures. The virus was Semliki Forest Virus, a group A arbovirus. It is apparent that between 20 and 80% inhibition of virus growth there is indeed the linear relationship discussed above between the interferon concentration and the virus inhibition.

It is important in an interferon assay to specify the virus and cell type, as was done in the legend to Fig. 2. Other factors, however, are also critical in influencing interferon assays. It is important to expose the particular cells employed to interferons for enough time to induce maximal antiviral activity. Usually this is accomplished by exposing cells to interferons overnight; that is, at least 14 hr, depending, of course, on how late you work. That enough incubation time has been allowed should be specifically checked, however, as the time to develop maximal activity varies in different systems.

The multiplicity of virus challenge is also important. Most effective interferon assays use a virus-to-cell ratio of 0.1:5.0. If the multiplicity of virus is too low, endogenous interferon production may become a factor in the assay. On the other hand, with high multiplicities of virus in some systems, the antiviral effect of the interferon is to some extent reversed. This is especially true when protection against viral cytopathic effect (CPE) is the end point being used in the assay, since CPE can occur in the absence of replication at high multiplicities of infection with some viruses.

Several other factors should be considered in interferon assays. After exposure of cells to an interferon preparation, the cultures should be washed at least twice. This is because many nonspecific inhibitors of virus replication are present in fluids sometimes used for interferon assays; this is especially true of serum samples. Washing cells usually eliminates these as antiviral factors. Also, in reading interferon assays, early is better; that is, more accurate titers are found with an early reading of viral CPE. This is due to multiple factors such as recovery of cells from interferon effects and the slow development of virus cytopathology even in interferon-treated cells. Finally, the age of cultures can be an important factor in interferon assays. Aging some types of cells in culture can increase the sensitivity of the cells to interferon action.

SPECIFIC ASSAYS FOR INTERFERONS AND INTERFERON STANDARDS (TABLE III)

The simplest and often the most convenient assay for interferons is based on protection against viral CPE. Cells are incubated with dilutions of putative interferon preparation, then infected with a virus, and later examined for virus CPE. The reciprocal of the greatest dilution of the interferon preparation that protects against virus infection is the titer of that preparation. In some laboratories the degree of CPE is quantitated by estimating the uptake of a vital dye. Many other assays are based on inhibition of viral CPE by interferon treatment. Plaque-reduction assays, for instance, have been employed to assay interferons for many years.

Another form of assay is the virus yield reduction and variations on it. The simplest application of this assay is the inhibition of yields of infectious virus. Cells are treated with an interferon and infected with virus; then at the end of a virus growth cycle, the culture fluids are titrated for yield of infectious virus. The data

TABLE III. Assays for Interferon

I. Inhibition of cytopathic effect
   A. Measured by direct microscopic examination of infected cells
   B. Vital dye uptake inhibition
II. Reduction in virus plaque formation
III. Reduction in virus yield
   Inhibition of
   A. Infectious virus
   B. Hemagglutinin
   C. Neuraminidase
   D. Viral RNA synthesis (radiochemically determined)
   E. Viral reverse transcriptase

shown in Fig. 2 are the result of a yield reduction assay. Variations on the yield reduction assay are legion, since theoretically the assay can be for any viral constituent or product. In fact, the first assays for interferon by Isaacs and Lindenmann were based on the inhibition of the yields of influenza virus hemagglutinin. Yields of viral neuraminidase have also served as assays for interferons.

The variety of such assays is limited only by the number of viral products known and the imagination of the investigator (Table III). For instance, in the presence of actinomycin D to inhibit host RNA synthesis, interferon-treated, virus-infected cells may be incubated with radioactive precursors to RNA (such as uridine). The amount of the precursor incorporated in viral RNA is then estimated, usually in a scintillation spectrometer. The reduction in RNA synthesis is related to the interferon concentration with which the cells had been treated. One other assay for interferon action employs the reverse transcriptase present in RNA tumor viruses. This is a sufficiently active enzyme to serve as a basis for an assay. Again the reduction in reverse transcriptase is proportional to the concentration of the interferon.

How can the results of such biological assays be compared in different laboratories that use different viruses, cells, and methods in their studies? The current method is to employ international standards for interferons; such standards are available for mouse interferon and for human fibroblast or leukocyte interferons among others. Their use is simple: samples of the international standard should be obtained and carefully titered against a laboratory standard. The titer of the international standard is supplied with the sample. When the laboratory standard is then quantitated in terms of international standard, the former is used in all future interferon assays. The results obtained in a given assay are then reported in terms of international units.

Let us take an example of the results obtained in a typical recent assay for viral CPE in my laboratory: it was found that it required 3 international units (IU) of mouse interferon to protect our line of L cells against the CPE of encephalomyocarditis (EMC) virus infection at a virus-to-cell multiplicity of 1. In the same assay a 1:8 dilution of a mouse serum thought to contain interferon protected the cells against CPE by EMC virus. The titer of interferon in the serum sample was therefore reported as 24 IU/ml of mouse interferon.

Now it may be, as mentioned earlier, that assays for quantitating interferons in other ways will soon be available. Radioimmunoassays, new assays based directly on the effects of interferons on cells such as reductions in particular viral or cellular enzymes, or effects on cell growth or the immune system are among such possibilities; these assays may well be more accurate, rapid, and repeatable than the biological assays used now. As mentioned, however, it will be very surprising if they are more sensitive than the latter.

DETAILS OF A RAPID BIOLOGICAL ASSAY FOR INTERFERONS

A simple, rapid assay for interferons is the CPE assay in microtiter plates. Microtiter plates are 96-well plastic tissue culture carriers (8 × 12 wells) in which each well takes about 0.25 ml of fluid. They may be obtained from any one of several manufacturers of plastic tissue culture ware.

The assay is started by adding 0.2 ml of the highest concentration of interferon to be tested to the first well. The other wells are filled with 0.1 ml of virus dilution medium; 0.1 ml of each dilution is then transferred serially to the next well. After mixing, 0.1 ml is passed in turn to the next well until the end of the dilution series is reached. The transfers may be made individually or with an eight-channel Titertek microtitrator, a multichannel pipette that can be very useful for such assays; it can be obtained from Flow Laboratories, Rockville, Maryland 20852.

Once the dilutions of interferon are completed, the cells to be tested are added to the microtiter dish. About 10,000 cells per well constitute a convenient number for a test. As a practical matter, I usually trypsin-treat a 75–100 cm^2 flask containing a semiconfluent monolayer of cell (about 10^7 cells) and suspend the cells in 50–100 ml of medium. Then 0.1 ml of this cell suspension is added to each well of the microtiter dish.

It is important to remember to include in each assay untreated cells to serve as virus controls (cells not treated with interferon and later virus infected) and cell controls (cells treated or not treated with interferon but not infected with virus to serve as toxicity controls). In addition, dilutions of the laboratory interferon standard should be added to each assay so that the results can be reported in terms of the international reference standard for the type of interferon being tested. Information about international reference standards may be obtained from the Research Resources Branch, Extramural Activities Program, NIAID, NIH, Bethesda, Maryland 20205.

After the interferon dilutions, the controls, and lab interferon standards have been incubated with the cells for 14 hr (overnight), the fluids are removed from the cells and the cells washed two to three times. The cells are then infected with a test virus at a low virus-to-cell multiplicity. In my laboratory, we employ a virus-to-cell ratio of 1:1. The test virus used is either the Indiana strain of vesicular stomatitis virus (VSV) or the encephalomyocarditis virus (EMC). Both virsues infect a broad range of cells and are rapidly cytopathic at a multiplicity of infection of 1. Distinct CPE is usually seen in less than 24 hr so that the virus can be conveniently added on one day and the assay read in an inverted microscope the next day.

The sensitivity of VSV or EMC to interferons in different cell systems varies, so that both viruses should be tested in order to arrive at the most sensitive assay. The viruses may be obtained from The American Type Culture Collection, 12301 Parklawn Drive, Rockville, Maryland 20852.

The results are interpreted in terms of the laboratory interferon reference standard as described earlier.

BIBLIOGRAPHY

Finter, N. B. (1978). The precision and comparative sensitivity of interferon assays. *Tex. Rep. Biol. Med.* **35,** 161–166.

Finter, N. B. (1973). The assay and standardization of interferon and interferon inducers. *In* "Interferons and Interferon Inducers" (N. B. Finter, ed). Amer. Elsevier, New York.

3

PURIFICATION AND PROPERTIES OF INTERFERONS

The purification of interferons has been a perplexing problem for many years. The probable cause of this is that interferons have very high biological activities; therefore, even amounts having a great deal of antiviral activity contain extremely small amounts of protein. Such a situation is the bane of the life of the protein chemist, as small amounts of protein are easily inactivated in various ways. Luckily, both the interferon molecule and the people who had been attempting to purify it had an inherent toughness. At present, several forms of human and mouse interferons have been purified. Amino acid sequence analysis was carried out on these.

PURIFICATION OF MOUSE AND HUMAN INTERFERONS

Almost every method of protein separation that has been discovered has been employed on the problem of interferon purification since Isaacs' original paper. The methods that have proved successful are actually rather simple, but the difficulties of many investigators leading up to these successes would be hard to catalogue.

The interferons that have been so far purified are two types of human interferons, alpha and beta, and the corresponding

TABLE IV. Old and New Nomenclature for Human and Mouse Interferons

New nomenclature	Old nomenclature	
	Human	Mouse
IFN-alpha	Le (leukocyte), type I, pH 2 stable	F (fast), C, type I, pH 2 stable
IFN-beta	F (fibroblast) Fi, type I, pH 2 stable	S (slow), A, B, type I, pH 2 stable
IFN-gamma	IIF (immune), type II, T, pH 2 labile, antigen-induced, mitogen-induced	IIF (immune), type 2, pH 2 labile, T, antigen-induced, mitogen-induced

mouse interferons. Several types of interferon have been discovered in several species; for a comparison of the old and the suggested new nomenclatures of these interferons, see Table IV. In humans, for instance, three types of interferons have so far been described (Table V). Type beta interferon is the only interferon produced by diploid human fibroblasts that have been stimulated with an interferon inducer such as the double-stranded RNA (dsRNA) polyinosinic:polycytidylic acid (polyIC). It is also produced, but not exclusively, when fibroblasts are infected with a

TABLE V. Types of Human Interferons

Type	Produced by	Inducer (approximate % of interferon produced)
Alpha	Fibroblasts	dsRNA (none)
	Fibroblasts	Virus (0–20%)
	Leukocytes	Virus (more than 99%)
	Lymphoblastoid cells	Virus (80%)
Beta	Fibroblasts	dsRNA (100%)
	Fibroblasts	Virus (80–100%)
	Leukocytes	Virus (less than 1%)
	Lymphoblastoid cells	Virus (20%)
Gamma	T lymphocytes	Mitogens (100%)
	T lymphocytes	Antigens (100%)

virus. A smaller percentage of the produced interferon is of the beta type, when leukocytes or lymphoblastoid cells are infected with viruses.

Alpha interferon is the major species of interferon produced when leukocytes are infected with virus. It is also produced by virus-infected lymphoblastoid cells and by fibroblasts. Alpha interferon has not so far been reported to be produced in cells induced to make interferon by dsRNA.

For the sake of completeness, type gamma interferon is included in Table V. It is produced under very special circumstances by T cells, but as of this writing has not yet been purified to the extent of the alpha and beta human interferons.

Human beta interferon from polyIC-treated human fibroblasts has been purified to homogeneity by a simple procedure involving blue sepharose chromatography and polyacrylamide gel electrophoresis. It has a molecular weight of 22,000–26,000 and a specific activity of 2–8 $\times$ 10^8 IU/mg of protein. Human alpha-type interferon has been purified from lymphoblastoid cell interferon by a combination of precipitation with trichloroacetic acid, antibody affinity, and SP-Sephadex chromatography, and polyacrylamide gel electrophoresis. It has a molecular weight of 18,500–22,000 and a specific activity of 2.2–2.5 $\times$ 10^8 units/mg of protein.

Several types of mouse interferons have also been purified. For instance, Erlich ascites cells stimulated by virus produce interferons of three molecular weight species. The mixture of interferons produced was first concentrated on controlled pore glass and then chromatographed on CM-Sephadex and phosphocellulose. Three active fractions resulted from these procedures; they were further purified on octyl sepharose and subjected to preparative isoelectric focusing and polyacrlyamide gel electrophoresis. These procedures yielded mouse interferons of molecular weights 35,000–40,000, 26,000–33,000, and 20,000. The first two are beta interferons; the last is an alpha interferon. Each of these interferons has a specific activity of about 2 $\times$ 10^9 units/mg of protein (Table VI).

The amino acid compositions of the interferons so far purified have been unremarkable. The amino acid sequences starting

TABLE VI. Properties of Purified Interferons

Type	Molecular weight	Specific activity of best available preparations (units per mg protein)
Human		
Alpha	18,500–22,000	$2.2–2.5 \times 10^8$
Beta	22,000–26,000	$2.0–8.0 \times 10^8$
Gamma	65,000–70,000	3×10^6
Gamma	40,000–46,000	3×10^6
Mouse		
Alpha	20,000	2×10^9
Beta	35,000–40,000	2×10^9
Beta	26,000–33,000	2×10^9
Gamma	70,000–90,000	more than 3×10^6
Gamma	40,000	more than 2×10^6

from the *N*-terminal end of these interferons is presently being worked out from purified interferons. The first 13 amino acids of mouse and human beta interferons and the first 20 of mouse and human alpha interferons have been published at the time of this writing (Fig. 3). Interestingly, mouse and human beta interferons are homologous at sites 3, 6, and 11; the homology between mouse and human alpha interferons is, however, much more extensive. Some of the cross-reactivity noted between human and

(A) Mouse interferons beta

                                    10

H-Ile-Asn-Tyr-Lys-Gln-Leu-Gln-Leu-Gln-Glu-Arg-Thr-Asn

Human beta interferon

                                    10

H-Met-Ser-Tyr-Asn-Leu-Leu-Gly-Phe-Leu-Gln-Arg-Ser-Ser

(B) Mouse interferon alpha

                                    10

H-Ala-Asp-Leu-Pro-Gln-Thr-Thr-Asn-Leu-Gly-Asn-Tys-Gly-Ala-Leu-Tys-Val-Leu-

      20

Leu-Ala-Gln

Human interferon alpha

                                    10

H-Ser-Asp-Leu-Pro-Gln-Thr-His-Ser-Leu-Gly-Asn-Arg-Arg-Ala-Leu-Ile-Leu-

      20

Leu-Ala-Gln

Fig. 3. Comparison of amino terminal sequences of purified mouse and human interferons.

mouse alpha interferons may be due to this homology; indeed, a similar homology may be the basis for the reported cross-species activity of human alpha interferon with rabbit, bovine, pig, and cat cells. All such cross-species reactivities will probably have their origins in structural homologies between interferons of widely differing animal species. This argues for some evolutionary preservation of the chemical structures.

Rapid progress in cloning the interferon gene has, however, overtaken and passed studies of the amino acid sequence of purified interferons. The complete amino acid sequences of human alpha and beta interferons has been deduced from the human genes responsible for their production that have been cloned in bacteria. There is much more homology between the human alpha and beta interferons than was suggested by their N-terminal sequences and immunological heterogeneity.

PROPERTIES OF INTERFERONS

Some interferons are glycoproteins. Their biological activities are therefore destroyed by proteolytic enzymes, but not by nucleases. It is not entirely clear what function the carbohydrates on interferons serve. Interferons without carbohydrates preserve much or all of their antigenicity, and biological activity when tested in tissue culture system, although they are of course smaller than natural interferons. Interestingly, the change heterogeneity of natural interferons that isoelectrically focus over a fairly wide range is lost when the sugar groups are removed.

The biological activities of alpha and beta interferons are stable to a wide pH range, from 2 to 11, and to heating to 56° for 30 min. An important exception here is the gamma interferons. Their biological activities are characteristically much more sensitive to acidity than are those of alpha and beta interferons. The gamma interferons also lose their biological activity when exposed to ionic detergents (such as sodium dodecyl sulfate) and to beta mercaptoethanol; of the other interferons, alpha is completely stable to such treatment and type beta is partially stable.

The most impressive characteristic of interferons to me, however, is their very great biological activity. To digress on this for a moment, the specific activity of mouse alpha and beta interferons ranged from 2×10^8 to 2×10^9 units/mg of protein. For the mouse interferons this means that one unit contains as little as 0.4 pg (or less than 10^{-12}gm) or 10^7 molecules. Since one unit of interferon in 1 ml of medium can protect more than 10^6 cells, the activity of interferons under these conditions approaches one molecule per cell. Interferons are, therefore, active at a concentration of about 10^{-15} M. This is lower than the effective concentration of many other highly active biological substances.

The multiple biological effects of interferons (Table VII) have all been reported to reside in a single molecule. This is likely only if, like a hormone, interferons cause multiple biological effects through some intermediary mechanism or mechanisms.

There is one final characteristic of interferons that should be mentioned: interferons are antigenic. Each of the three human interferons discussed earlier, for instance, is antigenically distinct; indeed, interferons may be purified by employing specific antisera. Antibodies to interferons are presently of great use in determining the biological role of interferons in various situations. However, animals do not produce antibodies to their own interferons. The classification of interferons advanced in Table IV is for the most part based on the antigenicities of the various interferons so far investigated. Indeed, until such time as the amino acids sequence of more interferons is known, we shall have to depend on antisera to classify interferons.

TABLE VII. Multiple Biological Effects of Purified Interferons

---

Antiviral activity

Inhibition of cell (and tumor) growth

Modulation of immune responses

Increased expression of histocompatibility antigens

Enhancement of sensitivity to toxicity of dsRNA forms

Enhancement of interferon production

Induction of some intracellular enzymes (e.g., oligo A synthetase, kinase)

Inhibition of some enzyme activities (e.g., ornithine decarboxylase)

BIBLIOGRAPHY

Gresser, I., DeMaeyer-Guignard, J., *et al.* (1979). Electrophoretically pure mouse interferon exerts multiple biologic effects. *Proc. Nat. Acad. Sci. USA* **76,** 5308–5312.

Knight E., Jr., Hunkapiller, M. W., *et al.* (1980). Human fibroblast interferon: Amino acid analysis and amino terminal amino acid sequence. *Science* **207,** 525–526.

Taira, H., Broeze, R. J., *et al.* (1980). Mouse interferons: amino terminal amino acid sequences of various species. *Science* **207,** 528–529.

Zoon, K. C., Smith, M. E., *et al.* (1980). Amino terminal sequence of the major component of human lymphoblastoid interferon. *Science* **207,** 527.

4

PRODUCTION OF INTERFERONS

Interferon production is usually an induced activity; in only a few cell types are interferons produced spontaneously. Thus the study of interferon induction provides some insights into the basic processes of induction of protein synthesis in animal cell systems. Because of the great biological activity of interferons, moreover, interferon messenger RNA can be assayed, thus making our insight into the induction of interferon more complete. Furthermore, the production of interferons is under a tight cellular control mechanism, so that some understanding of such mechanisms has been obtained through the study of interferon production.

Several practical problems arise in the study of interferon production. Such a variety of substances induces interferons in cell culture systems and in animals that there is little to go on in trying to form a unified hypothesis about what sort of chemical structure is responsible for interferon induction. It would be useful to have such information in order to design more active and less toxic interferon inducers. It is also uncertain whether interferon inducers must enter the cell to be active.

Another problem relates to the quantity of interferons currently available. Only very small amounts are made by animal cells, but its therapeutic use requires much larger quantities than are currently available. One important question is how to satisfy this need in a manner that is economically feasible. Two general solutions are possible. The first is to produce large quantities of interferon and use them therapeutically; this might be referred to as the exogenous approach. The other solution is to induce humans to make their own interferon, an endogenous approach. The exogenous approach requires very large stocks of interferon; the endogenous approach requires a nontoxic, effective inducer that can be repeatedly used.

INTERFERON INDUCERS

As can be seen in Table VIII there is indeed a variety of agents that induce interferons. They have little in common chemically or structurally. It therefore seems that interferon induction is a response to a number of stimuli and is not dependent on a paticular chemical structure.

The first group of interferon inducers described was, of course, viruses. Almost every animal virus under the right conditions can act as an interferon inducer. Single- or double-stranded RNA or DNA viruses all induce interferons; usually active virus is used, but heat- or UV-inactivated viruses under some conditions can induce high interferon titers. Some groups of viruses, however, tend to be good inducers of interferon in almost all situations tested; therefore, these are the ones that are generally

TABLE VIII. Classes of Interferon Inducers

  I. Animal viruses, active or inactivated
 II. Nonviral inducers, natural products
     A. Bacteria or bacterial products
     B. Bacteriophage
     C. Chlamydiae
     D. Rickettsiae
     E. Mycoplasma
     F. Protozoa
     G. Fungi or fungal extracts
III. Nonviral inducers, synthetic products
     A. Polynucleotides
     B. Anionic polymers
     C. Low-molecular-weight inducers
 IV. Inducers of gamma interferons
     A. Mitogens
     B. Antigens

employed. Paramyxoviruses, such as Newcastle disease virus (NDV) or Sendai virus, are favorites; a number of arboviruses are also excellent inducers, although they are often less readily available than NDV or Sendai virus.

In the early days of studies on interferons, when viruses were the only known inducers, it was easy to speculate on what exactly an interferon inducer was, that is, whether there was a specific chemical structure involved in interferon induction. When it was discovered that some forms of double-stranded RNA were also excellent interferon inducers, there was a notion that viruses could induce interferon production because they formed species of double-stranded RNA during the course of their replication. This is probably not the only explanation for interferon induction by viruses, as studies with virus mutants do not necessarily confirm this notion. Moreover, as is discussed later, interferons are induced by a large variety of substances that seem to have nothing at all to do with double-stranded RNA.

The first nonviral interferon inducer discovered was endotoxin from *Escherichia coli*. Soon after that a number of other substances were found, including other endotoxins and other bacterial products such as lipids, lipopolysaccharides, capsular polysaccharides, and even toxoid from *Corynebacterium diphtheriae*. As might be expected, numerous intact bacteria also induce interferon production. Most of these organisms grow intracellularly.

Once the cat was out of the bag that nonviral inducers were possible, a large variety of biological substances were found to induce interferon production. T4 phage and double-stranded RNA forms from the replication of RNA phages were found to be inducers. A large variety of organisms from other groups are also active. Among the Chlamydiae, the trachoma and psittacosis agents induce interferon, as do a number of rickettsiae and several mycoplasma. Even intracellular parasites such as *Plasmodium berghei*, *Toxoplasmic gondii*, and *Trypanasoma cruzi* induce interferon production.

Perhaps the most interesting of the interferon inducers are the products from fungi or fungal extracts. These are probably all related to the killer double-stranded RNA forms carried by many species of yeast. In fact, as far back as 1953, Shope reported that an extract of *P. funiculosum* that he called Helenine was an antiviral substance. In investigating the mechanism of action of Helenine, it was discovered that the active component was a form of double-stranded RNA present in yeast. This discovery led to the synthesis of one of the most active of the synthetic, nonviral inducers of interferons, the ribopolynucleotides.

The most commonly studied of these is the homopolymer ribonucleotide pair polyriboinosinic:polyribocytidylic acid (polyIC). This is the standard compound against which all other synthetic inducers of interferon are measured. Other polymers that are at least somewhat active are single-stranded homoribopolymers such as polyriboinosinic acid (polyrI), alternating copolymers (polyrI•rC:polyrA•rU) or combinations of homopolymers and copolymers (polyrI•polyrC-rG). In addition, at least one polydeoxyribonucleotide, polydA•dT, has been reported to be an active interferon inducer.

Several chemical modifications in polyIC, or another active homoribopolymer pair, polyAU, have yielded a number of good inducers of interferon. The primary molecular alterations include (Fig. 4) replacement of the hydrogen at position 5 of cytosine with —Br in polyIC, or with halogens or —CH$_3$ in the uridine of polyAU. The 2' hydroxyl group can be modified by replacement with —H, —OCH$_3$ in polyIC or by —N$_3$ or F in polyAU. The oxygen at the 2 position of the cytosine in polyIC can be replaced by a sulfur group; finally, the nitrogen in position 7 of the purine of polyAU or polyIC can be replaced by a —CH group. Unfortunately, none of these modifications has yielded an interferon inducer that is so greatly superior to polyIC that it has been clinically useful.

Chemical modifications of polyIC are carried out for two basic reasons. PolyIC itself and unfortunately all of its interferon-inducing modified forms are quite toxic for animals. In addition, there are nucleases present in humans and animals that can attack double-stranded forms of RNA. Chemical modifications of polyIC that increase its ability to induce interferon often increase

29

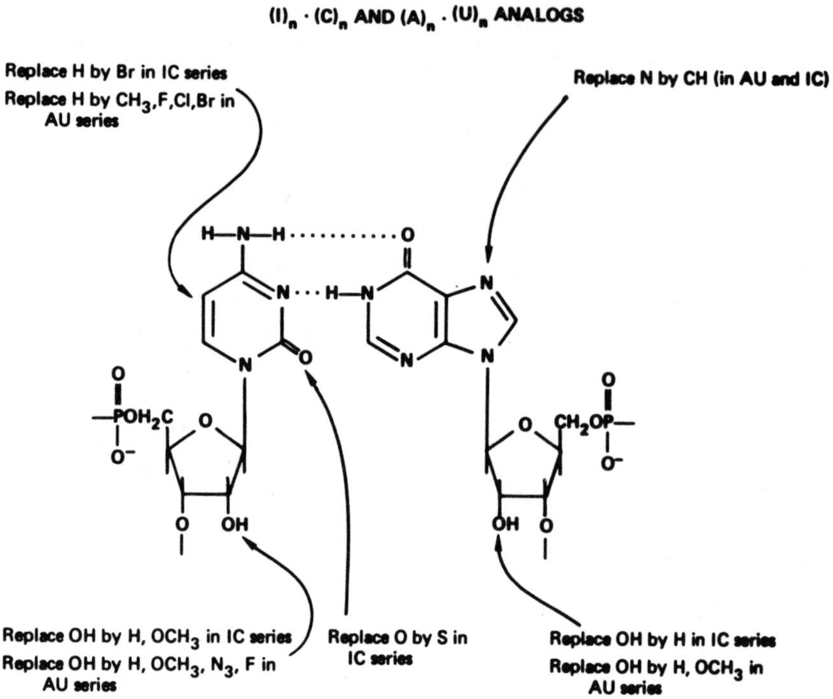

$(I)_n \cdot (C)_n$ AND $(A)_n \cdot (U)_n$ ANALOGS

Replace H by Br in IC series
Replace H by CH$_3$,F,Cl,Br in AU series

Replace N by CH (in AU and IC)

Replace OH by H, OCH$_3$ in IC series
Replace OH by H, OCH$_3$, N$_3$, F in AU series

Replace O by S in IC series

Replace OH by H in IC series
Replace OH by H, OCH$_3$ in AU series

Fig. 4. Chemical modifications of polyinsinic acid:polycytidylic acid (polyIC) or polyadenylic acid:polyurydylic acid (polyAU).

The molecules are pictured as base-paired I and C or A and U. Going clockwise from the upper left, the hydrogen at position 5 of the cytosine may be replaced by a bromide (Br) in polyIC or with fluoride (F), chloride (Cl), or a methyl (—CH$_3$) group, in AU.

The nitrogen at position 7 of the purine in AU or IC can be replaced by a —CH group. The 2'-hydroxyl group of the purine can be replaced by an —H group in IC, and in the AU series, by an —H or —OCH$_3$; the oxygen at position 2 of the cytosine in IC can be replaced by a sulfur(S) group; and the 2' hydroxyl group of the pyrimidine ribose can be replaced by a hydrogen (H) or —OCH$_3$ group in the IC series, and by either of these or by N$_3$ or F in AU. (Based on data provided by Dr. Paul Torrence, NIAMDD, NIH.)

the toxicity of the molecule. Sometimes the sensitivity to nucleases is decreased.

One significant improvement in polyIC as an interferon inducer is attained by its aggregation with other molecules that appear to protect the RNA from nucleases. At least two of these have been advanced as interferon inducers with clinical potential:

polyIC + DEAE-dextran, or polyIC•poly-L-lysine, coprecipitated with carboxymethylcellulose. Both resist attack by nucleases; the latter combination molecule has been able to induce interferon production in species of monkeys in which there has been no reported interferon induction with polyIC. Clinical testing of polyIC•poly-L-lysine is in progress; it will be important to follow these studies to see whether interferon inducers have a future as clinical tools. As noted earlier, however, other chemical modifications of polyIC such as insertion of sulfur for oxygen (thiophosphate analogues), also resist nuclease attack; this resistance certainly may account for their improved ability to induce interferon. As mentioned earlier, the usefulness of such a compound is limited by the increase in animal toxicity that appears to go hand in hand with increased ability to induce interferon synthesis.

In addition to the double-stranded RNA forms several anionic polymers have been reported to induce interferon in animals. These include pyran copolymers, polyacrylic and polymethacrylic acids, and polyacrylic acid–poly-allylsucrose. Other anionic polymers that induce interferon synthesis are polyvinyl sulfate and dextran phosphate.

A number of low-molecular-weight interferon inducers have been reported. Tilorone (bisdiethylaminoethyl fluorenone) induces interferon synthesis in mice, but alas, not in humans. The dyes acridine and quinacrine also induce interferon in animals. Finally, to complete the list of active small molecules, propanediamine, a quinoline compound (BL-20803), a furan (MA-56), the radioprotective mercaptoalkylamine AET, and a substituted pyrimidine all induce interferon in animals and in some cases in tissue cultures.

To summarize, many interferon inducers have been reported. Because of their diverse chemical and structural nature, it is impossible at present to pick out a specific interferon-inducing molecular structure. Interferon inducers do not appear to hold much promise as clinically useful compounds, partially because of their high toxicity in animals. In addition, hyporesponsiveness to these inducers follows their administration (see the following discussion).

MECHANISMS OF INTERFERON PRODUCTION

The production of beta interferon in human fibroblasts appears to be controlled by a gene on chromosome number 9. In fact, studies with chromosome translocations have identified the short arm of chromosome 9 as the locus of the interferon production gene; however, some studies have suggested other chromosomal loci for beta interferon production (chromosomes 2 and 5). Additional hybrid-cell line studies have indicated that monkey interferon production is correlated with the presence of monkey chromosome 22. So far human interferons other than type beta have not been identified with specific chromosomal loci.

The control over interferon production is quite complex, as will become apparent as this section develops. For instance, at least four gene loci were involved in *in vivo* production of interferons in mice; they were related to the virus used as an inducer (Table IX). If-1, which is linked to a minor histocompatability antigen, H-28, is the best studied of these. There appear to be only two alleles for the If-1 locus: If^h, for high interferon production, and If^l, for low. The prototypes of mouse strains studied for If-1 are C57BL (If^h) and BALB/c (If^l). If-1 is associated with production of alpha and beta interferons by hematopoetic cells, lymphocytes, and macrophages. What seems most surprising about this system is that four different loci should be concerned with interferon production induced by various viruses. Why should the locus for interferon production by the paramyxovirus NDV differ from that of another member of the same group, Sendai virus? Why should the various loci exist for control of what appears to be the same interferon product? It seems clear that study of the

TABLE IX. Gene Loci Involved in Production of Serum Interferon in Inbred Mouse Strains

Viral inducer	Number of loci involved	Designation
Newcastle disease virus	1	If-1
Mouse mammary tumor virus	1	If-2
Sendai virus	2	If-3 and If-4

genetics of interferon production may answer many questions about gene organization and control in animals. It is certainly possible that many more forms of interferons exist than we are presently aware of and that each form has a distinct gene.

Figure 5 is an example of production of interferon in response to virus infection in tissue culture. These results are taken from studies of primary chick cells infected with a group A arbovirus, Semliki Forest virus. They are somewhat atypical in that interferon production is a bit late with respect to virus replication; interferon production induced by polyIC begins within 2 hr of addition of the inducer.

The production of interferons (Fig. 5) has an induction phase of several hours in which the inducer binding, uptake, and processing must take place. The interferon gene then must be derepressed because an interferon is usually an induced protein (there are, however, unusual cell types where it is constitutive). Studies on superinduction, discussed later, further suggest that a repressor for interferon production normally is produced. The actual production phase of an interferon involves transcription of interferon

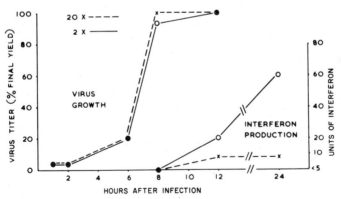

Fig. 5. Induction of interferon production by virus.
Chick embryo fibroblast (CEF) monolayers were infected by Semliki Forest virus (SFV) at virus-to-cell multiplicities of 2:1 or 20:1. At the indicated times after infection, cells were frozen. After thawing monolayer samples of tissue, the culture fluids were assayed for virus and the results plotted as a percentage of the maximum titer reached, which was taken as 100%. The balance of the culture fluids were treated with acid (pH 2) to inactivate the SFV. CEF interferon is stable to such acid pHs. The fluids were then neutralized and assayed for interferon.

mRNA, its translation, posttranscriptional processing of interferon, and, finally, secretion of interferon into the extracellular fluid. Because of the extremely high biological activity of interferons and their ready identification, interferon production is probably one of the best-studied induced activities in animal cells.

One aspect of interferon production not explicit in Fig. 5 is that control over it is quickly reasserted after the induction process is over, so that interferon production declines rapidly in cells that survive the effects of the interferon inducer. Another point (which Fig. 5 does illustrate) is that the level of interferon produced varies with the multiplicity of virus infection, if, like SFV in this system, the virus shuts off cell protein synthesis (and, therefore, interferon production) during the course of its growth cycle.

In *in vivo* studies some substances induce early interferon production from 2 to 8 hr after addition of the inducer. These early inducers include polyIC and bacteria or bacterial products. Late inducers take 6–16 hr to induce interferon production and include most viruses, tilorone, and the several anionic polymers. Production of gamma interferons in T cells after induction with antigens or mitogens is a much slower process, taking from 3 days for phytohemagglutinin to 7 days for poke weed mitogen.

Understanding of the biological aspects of interferon induction has been facilitated by remarkably sensitive assays for interferon mRNA. In devising these assays, two properties of interferon have been exploited. The first is interferon's high specific activity. This has made possible the detection of the minute amounts of interferon that may be stimulated by exceedingly small quantities of interferon messenger RNA. The second is the species specificity of interferons. This has made possible unequivocal identification of an interferon as the specific product of a messenger RNA.

Interferon messenger RNAs are 9–12S RNA forms when sedimented in sucrose gradients (Fig. 6). The first experiments to assay for interferon messenger RNA employed incubation of the putative messenger with heterologous cells (Table X). The culture medium was later tested for activity of an interferon of the species from which the interferon messenger RNA had been extracted.

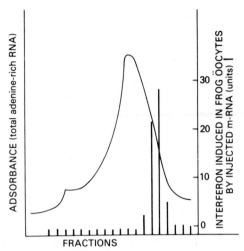

Fig. 6. Interferon messenger RNA-fractionation of adenylic acid (A)-rich RNA on sucrose gradients and its frog oocyte injection.

Namalva lymphoblastoid cells were induced to make interferons by infection with Newcastle disease virus. After about 14 hr the cells were removed from culture and washed. The cellular RNA was extracted and the adenylic acid-rich fraction separated by chromatography. This yielded a preparation with a high content of messenger RNA (mRNA) that was further purified and concentrated by alcohol precipitation. This mRNA preparation was then fractionated on a sucrose gradient (curved line) and the fractions monitored in a spectrophotometer for total RNA content. The top of the gradient is to the right. Sample of these fractions were then microinjected into frog oocytes. After overnight incubation of the oocytes, the fluid in which they were suspended was withdrawn and assayed for interferon content (vertical lines). It should be noted that the maximum interferon-inducing fractions sedimented more slowly than did the bulk of the messenger RNA. (Based on the results of several reports of interferon messenger RNA production and its activity in frog oocytes.)

For instance, after messenger RNA from virus or polyIC-induced mouse embryo cells had been incubated with chick cells, the medium was later found to contain mouse interferon. Injection of messenger RNA preparations into frog oocytes allows, however, some quantitation in such systems, so that this approach has been employed in several laboratories. Interestingly, as in cell cultures, the interferon produced by interferon messenger RNA injected frog oocytes is secreted into the medium. Finally, several types of cell-free systems translate interferon messenger RNA to form active interferon.

One of the chief uses of such assays for interferon messenger

TABLE X. Assay Methods for Interferon Messenger RNA[a]

A. Heterologous cells
B. *Xenopus laevis* oocytes
C. Cell free systems[b]

[a] Messenger RNA has been extracted from human, mouse, chick, and monkey cells induced with Newcastle disease virus or polyIC.

[b] Krebs II ascites, rabbit reticulocyte, Ehrlich ascites, and wheat germ cell-free systems have been employed.

RNA has been to study the production and fate of various messenger RNA forms. Generally, interferon messenger RNA is absent before induction; a few hours after addition of an inducer it rises, but later it declines and returns to undetectable levels. The amount of messenger RNA produced is roughly proportional to the amount of interferon made by the cells. There is one interesting exception to these findings, however. In lymploblastoid Namalva cells induced by NDV to make high titers of interferon, interferon messenger RNA was recovered from cells several hours after they had stopped producing interferon. This, together with data on superinduction of interferons (see the following discussion), suggests that more than one mechanism relating to control of interferon production exists.

Superinduction refers to a paradoxical enhancement of interferon production in cells treated with metabolic inhibitors. This phenomenon is not restricted to interferon induction, as it has been reported for enzymes such as tyrosine amino transferase. The general methodology employed is indicated in Fig. 7. After cells were stimulated to produce interferon with polyIC, but before interferon was made, a reversible inhibitor of protein synthesis such as cycloheximide was added to the medium during the first few hours of the incubation. Slightly before the time the inhibitor of protein synthesis was washed off, an inhibitor of RNA synthesis such as actinomycin D was added. Another inhibitor of mRNA synthesis, 5,6-dichloro-1-β-D-ribofuranosylbenzimidazole (DRB), can be added; unlike actinomycin D, the action of DRB is reversible. As can be seen in Fig. 7, under these conditions interferon production started later than usual, but reached much

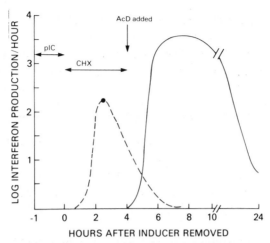

Fig. 7. Superinduction of beta interferon in human fibroblasts.
Human fibroblast monolayers were treated with polyIC for 1 hr, they were washed, and
then cycloheximide (CHX) was added for 4 hr. The cycloheximide was then removed by
washing and actinomycin D (AcD) was added to the cultures. Fluids were harvested hourly
and assayed for interferon content. The broken line represents control cultures treated with
polyIC, but not exposed to CHX or AcD. The interferon production in control cultures
was maximal by 2 hr after removal of the polyIC, whereas the maximal production in
superinduced cultures (those exposed to CHX and AcD) was later but persisted for a much
longer period of time. (Based on several reports on superinduction of interferon in human
fibroblasts.)

higher levels and went on for longer; indeed, because of this later
shut-off, 20–100 times as much interferon was produced in
superinduced cells as in normally induced ones.

The status of interferon messenger RNA under superinduction conditions is of great interest. Several studies have indicated
that the half-life of interferon messenger RNA is increased at least
three- to fourfold in superinduced cells. These results suggest that
normally interferon is not produced because of the presence of a
repressor substance, probably a protein that acts on the interferon
messenger RNA. If interferon is to be induced, the repressor concentration has to be reduced below an effective level; while normal production is taking place, however, the level of repressor
quickly builds up again, interferon messenger RNA is degraded or
inactivated, and interferon production is halted. During the
superinduction process, it would appear that the production of

the repressor is delayed, so that the half-life of the interferon messenger RNA is significantly extended.

Several other important phenomena relating to control of interferon production have been reported. Priming refers to an increased production of interferon in cells treated with interferon before interferon induction. This is a property of the interferon molecule itself, as purified interferons prime for interferon production. In primed cells, interferon production is not only increased, but it also commences at an earlier time point than does interferon production in unprimed cells. Unlike superinduction, priming does not appear to be related to an increased half-life for interferon messenger RNA, but seems to be due to its very early production.

Hyporesponsiveness or blocking, on the other hand, refer to an inhibition of interferon production, following treatment with high concentrations of interferon. Also, repeated induction of interferon results in hyporesponsiveness. The mechanism for this phenomenon is not clear and its relationship to interferon action is dubious, since purified preparations of interferon do not have blocking activity.

The anatomical location for interferon production in the cell cytoplasm is the rough endoplasmic reticulum (RER). The nascent chains of interferon are probably glycosylated initially at their site of synthesis (Fig. 8). From the RER the newly formed interferon is passed on to the Golgi cisternae, also in the cytoplasm. The interferon finally ends up in secretory vesicles from which it enters the extracellular fluid. In these respects interferons resemble most other secreted glycoproteins.

Interferon production in animals has of course been extensively studied. As already indicated by the diverse genetic loci related to interferon induction by various substances (Table IX), interferon production is a complex phenomenon. The anatomic location of interferon production depends to a great extent on the inducer and its site of injection. Intravenous, intradermal, intracerebral, or intranasal injections of inducers give rise, respectively, to high interferon titers in the serum, the skin, the brain, or the lungs. As a virus spreads, the site of interferon production changes. For instance, intraperitoneal inoculation of encepha-

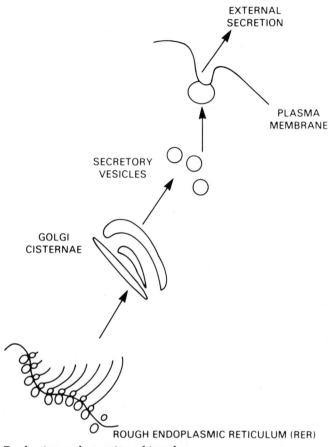

EXTERNAL
SECRETION

PLASMA
MEMBRANE

SECRETORY
VESICLES

GOLGI
CISTERNAE

ROUGH ENDOPLASMIC RETICULUM (RER)

Fig. 8. Production and secretion of interferons.
Interferon is synthesized on membrane-associated polyribosomes attached to the rough endoplasmic reticulum (RER). Figure 8 depicts elongating interferon molecules attached to smaller ribosomal subunits. Addition of carbohydrates is probably initiated on the nascent interferon molecules while they are still associated with the RER. The interferon is released into the Golgi cisternae where addition of carbohydrate is completed. Interferon is then transferred to secretory vesicles that migrate to the cell surface. When the secretory vesicles reach the plasma membrane, they fuse with it and release their content into the extracellular fluid. The interferon protein does not have to be glycosylated in order to be secreted by the cell.

lomycarditis virus gave rise to local production of interferon. When viremia occurred, interferon appeared in the serum, an interferonemia (Fig. 9); finally, as virus localized in the heart and central nervous system, interferon was found in these organs.

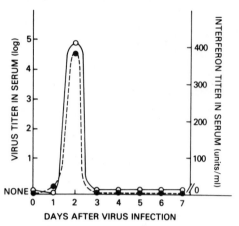

Fig. 9. Viremia and interferonemia after infection with encephalomyocarditis (EMC) virus in mice.

Mice were infected with 10–100 infectious units of EMC virus by intraperitoneal injection. The animals were bled each day for one week and the serum samples were titrated for levels of virus and interferon. Both virus (open circles) and interferon (closed circles) were found in the blood 48 hr after injection. (Based on the results of several studies on interferon production following virus infection in mice.)

Both viral and nonviral inducers have been employed to produce interferon in experimental animals and man. Whereas nonviral inducers such as endotoxin or polyIC gave rise to interferon production over a 2–8 hr period, viral induction usually took longer. This distinction may be artificial as viruses may have to initiate their replication, or at least be processed in some manner to induce interferon.

As mentioned previously, probably because of the presence of nucleases that are capable of hydrolyzing double-stranded RNA forms, polyIC is not an effective inducer in man and in some animals, but, when combined to form a polyIC–L lysine complex, high titers of interferon can be induced in previously recalcitrant species. Other inducers have problems related to species specificity; tilorone induces high titers of interferon in mice even when administered intragastrically but is inactive in other species.

A great deal of effort has gone into determining which types of cell or organs are involved in various *in vivo* studies of induction of interferons. The particular organ or cell type seems to vary with the inducer and its route of administration. The types of studies employed have included irradiation, organ removal (such as spleenectomy or thymectomy), use of antilymphocyte serum, or genetically unusual mouse strains, such as nude mice; however, no clear-cut picture of a single organ or cell type responsible for all interferon production has emerged from a mass of data, for it would seem that each system must be studied on its own.

One interesting phenomenon that may limit the use of *in vivo* interferon inducers (in addition to toxicity and nuclease problems) is hyporesponsiveness. This is probably analogous to the hyporesponsiveness or blocking seen in *in vivo* systems. In animals, repeated stimulation with an interferon inducer not only causes interferon to be produced but also results in a period of several days after interferon production has ceased, during which little or no interferon may be induced. This hyporesponsive period does not appear to be due to the antiviral action of interferon alone, since it may persist long after antiviral activity has diminished. Hyporesponsiveness could, of course, severely limit the possible effectiveness of interferon inducers. Interestingly, hyporesponsiveness may be transferred by a serum factor that is clearly not interferon, since it has no antiviral activity. Hyporesponsiveness in mice can, however, be overcome by administering prostoglandins at the same time as the interferon inducer. So far prostaglandins E_1, A_1, and F_1 alpha are effective in this respect. It is not at all clear at this time what hyporesponsiveness, serum hyporesponsive factor, or the effect of prostoglandins on them are.

The last problem discussed in this section is central to the future of the clinical use of interferon; that is, how can we obtain enough interferon to establish that it is a useful substance for treating human diseases, and, if interferon is useful, how can enough of it be made to satisfy the need arising from that utility? These are not easy problems because cells seem to produce so little interferon with respect to the large amounts required for clinical use.

There are realistically three basic methods that might be employed right now to increase interferon production: better applications of the methods we are now using, synthesis of human interferons or active fragments of them, and cloning of the human interferon gene with production of human interferons in microorganism.

The main methods currently used to produce interferons are stimulation by paramyxoviruses of white blood cells from the buffy coat of donated blood, or of lymphoblastoid cells to produce a mixture containing mostly alpha and some beta interferon, or superinduction of human fibroblast cultures with polyIC to produce beta-type interferon. There is not any particularly good method for producing human gamma interferon, but about the best system available is to stimulate human buffy coat cells with a mitogen. Almost all the interferon used so far in clinical studies has come from the first method descibed, the stimulation of human buffy coat white cells with paramyxoviruses; therefore, the interferon that has been primarily used is of the alpha type. There has been really only one consistently reliable source for this material, the laboratory of Dr. Kari Cantell in Helsinki, Finland, and only through his persistent efforts has there been some material available for the relatively small number of clinical studies that have been so far carried out.

Another possible source of supply is the stimulation of human lymphoblastoid cells to produce interferon. The Namalva line is a potential source of very high titers of human alpha and beta interferons; these cells can be grown in enormous amounts in very dense cultures. The only drawback to using this source of supply is that the cells originally came from a malignant tumor (a Burkitt lymphoma), so that the interferon they supply may have only limited use; however, if it can be shown that there is no trace of host or viral genetic material in these interferon preparations, they could certainly be considered for general use. The origin of Namalva cells should not *a priori* rule out the general use of the interferons they make. Indeed, limited clinical studies with this material are under way at present.

The other currently employed source of human interferons, beta interferon from human diploid fibroblast cultures superinduced by polyIC, has definite potential for greatly increasing yields of interferon. There are, however, in this procedure technical questions about how to grow large enough quantities of human diploid cells to satisfy the potential need for the interferon they produce. One problem is that diploid human cells cannot be grown in large-volume suspension cultures; the solution might be the growth of such cells on carriers that could be kept in suspension. One additional problem related to the use of human beta type interferon is that this interferon is "sticky." It tends to adhere to many types of columns, surfaces, etc., to which other sorts of interferons do not adhere; therefore, it tends to stay at its site of injection and not enter the circulation for distribution all over the body. The latter shortcoming might be overcome by purifying the beta interferon to the point where it could be inoculated intravenously.

The other methods to be discussed are at present theoretical, since they have so far provided no interferon for clinical use; however, they do possess the potential for providing very large amounts, perhaps more than enough to satisfy the needs for interferon, should it prove to be clinically useful.

Several different laboratories have recently worked out the amino acid sequence analysis of alpha and beta human interferons. Therefore, it might now be possible to synthesize interferon molecules that are active in humans. It might even be possible to synthesize active small fragments of some of the human interferons, if such could be found, as the technical problems involved in making a whole sequence of over 150 amino acids chemically might be at present insurmountable. In addition, it might be possible to synthesize DNA sequences capable of programming for production of the human interferons. These DNA forms could be inserted into microorganisms that would then act as sources for human interferons. Finally, the cloning of the human alpha and beta interferon genes may provide large quantities of clinically useful material.

The final possible source of human interferons is direct cloning of the human interferon gene. This is already accomplished, but it remains to be seen whether this feat will provide us with a useful source of human interferon. The method used was to extract polyadenylic acid-rich 12S RNA (messenger RNA) from human leukocytes induced to make interferon by Sendai virus. This RNA was used as a template for the synthesis of a double-stranded complementary DNA (cDNA) that was then inserted

TABLE XI. Cloning of Human Interferon Genes

1. Extract 12S fraction of poly-A-rich mRNA from human leukocytes induced to make IFN
2. IFN-mRNA used as template for synthesis of double-stranded cDNA
3. IFN-cDNA elongated with dCMP and joined to *E. coli* DNA
4. Screening of clones of *E. coli* for recombinant DNA hybridizing to IFN-mRNA
5. Checking positive clones for production of HuIFN-alpha

TABLE XII. Some Possible Methods of Increasing the Supply of Human Interferons

I. Expansion of currently used methods of production from:
    A. White cells of human donated blood
    B. Lymphoblastoid cells
    C. Superinduced diploid fibroblasts
II. Synthesis of human interferons
    A. Total synthesis of human IFN molecules
    B. Synthesis of active portions of human IFNs
    C. Synthesis of a DNA capable of programming for the production of human IFNs, and insertion of this into microorganisms
III. Cloning of human IFN genes

into *E. coli.* A large number of clones of this organism were screened for a recombinant DNA that could hybridize with the interferon messenger RNA. Several clones that produced human alpha interferon were found (Table XI). This methodology could theoretically be used for production of all three human interferon types.

The methods that might be employed to increase virus supply of human interferons are summarized in Table XII.

BIBLIOGRAPHY

Cavalieri, R. L., and Pestka, S. (1977). Synthesis of interferon in heterologous cells, cell-free extracts, and *Xenopus laevis* oocytes. *Tex. Rep. Biol. Med.* **35**, 117–125.

De Maeyer, E., and De Maeyer-Guignard, J. (1979). Considerations on mouse genes influencing interferon production and action. *Interferon* **1**, 75–100.

Epstein, L. B. (1977). Mitogen and antigen induction of interferon *in vivo* and *in vitro*. *Tex. Rep. Biol. Med.* **35**, 57–62.

Torrence, P. F., and DeClercq, E. (1977). Inducers and induction of interferons. *Pharmacol. Ther. Part A* **2**, 1–88.

5
MECHANISMS OF ANTIVIRAL ACTION

In order to understand what is known of the antiviral action of interferons, the reader must be acquainted with virus structure and function. What follows is a very brief review of the details of these stressing the aspects that are affected by interferon action.

THE STRUCTURE OF VIRUSES

Viruses may contain either RNA or DNA as their genetic material (genome). Every form of RNA or DNA has been found in some type of virus; single- or double-stranded DNA- or RNA-containing viruses have been described. Whatever the form of the viral genome is, however, it is protected by a protein-containing structure. This structure may be made up of one or several proteins. In addition to structural proteins, functional proteins are often present in viruses. These are enzymes; some of the virus-associated enzymes are related to the entry or exit of viruses from cells, whereas others catalyze the polymerization of viral nucleic acids. Whether or not a virus contains a structural polymerase is very much related to the nature of the viral genome. This will be discussed in the following section.

In addition to RNA or DNA and proteins, some viruses contain lipids in the forms of phospholipids, glycolipids, or cholesterol. These are present in DNA or RNA viruses that have an outer membrane as part of their structure. The membrane is a mosaic of viral proteins and lipids. It surrounds the virus, protects it from the environment, and is important in the adsorbtion of the virus to cell surfaces.

VIRUS REPLICATION

Whether or not a virus contains an outer membrane, however, the first step in its infectious cycle is adsorption to a cell. This fixes the virus to the cell surface long enough for the virus to penetrate the cell membrane, so that the viral genome enters the intracellular environment. Once penetration of the virus genome has taken place, at least partial uncoating follows in order for the viral RNA or DNA to function.

The function of a viral genome involves the synthesis of viral proteins and nucleic acids. The viral lipids are often incorporated from pool of preexisting cell lipids already present in the plasma membrane. If the viral genome consists of an RNA form that is able to act as a messenger RNA, i.e., able to induce the cells to make viral proteins directly (positive-stranded RNA), this is the first synthetic step in the replication process; the viral RNA is translated to produce a viral polymerase. The polymerase then uses the viral RNA of the infecting virus particles as a template to make more viral RNA. If, however, the viral genome is a species of RNA that does not act as a messenger RNA, that is, does not contain the genetic information for viral protein synthesis (negative-stranded RNA), in order to get started the virus must also have its own functional polymerase. This enzyme produces viral RNA in a manner similar to that of the polymerase induced by infection with positive-stranded viruses. The viral RNA made early in infection by the polymerase can be translated to produce viral proteins; i.e., it can act as a messenger RNA (mRNA).

In the case of infections with viruses that have a DNA genome, the virus must have its own DNA-directed RNA polymerase, or early in infection it must use a cellular polymerase.

Viral protein synthesis is very similar to cell-directed protein synthesis. Viral mRNA capable coding for virus protein synthesis attaches to a subunit of a cell organelle, the ribosome. In order to attach this ribosomal subunit, several proteins (initiation factors), guanosine triphosphate (GTP), and a form of amino acid transfer RNA—one of the species of transfer RNA (tRNA) for the amino acid methionine (Met-tRNA$_i$), must first interact with the viral mRNA. When this series of reactions is completed, the other subunit of the ribosome is added. The structure of the mRNA then determines the sequence of amino acid carrying tRNAs that attach to ribosomes as they come in contact with the viral mRNA. The tRNAs attached to the ribosomes determine the sequence of amino acids in the nascent protein. The sequence of amino acids is the most significant factor in providing the protein produced with its biological characteristics; that is, whether the protein will be structural or functional and what its exact nature will be. The virus of course directs the protein-synthetic machinery of the cell to produce viral proteins instead of cellular proteins.

The early course of viral infection is determined by the viral mRNA's and proteins that are produced. Later in infection other viral constituents may be made, depending on the nature of the virus. When the structural and functional constituents of the virus are formed, the virus assembles these. The assembly of the virus is primarily determined by the chemical structure of the viral constituents. It may take place wholly within the cytoplasm, in which case the virus must induce the cell to break open in order to release the progeny virus; in other cases, especially with viruses that have outer membranes as a structural unit, the virus assembles at the cell surface, the plasma membrane. In so doing, the virus gains egress from the cell by incorporating a modified segment of the plasma membrane and budding from the cell surface.

VIRUS EFFECTS ON CELLS

Viruses often have profound effects on the cells they have infected. The most obvious of these effects is the induction of severe damage or cytopathic effect (CPE), resulting finally in cell death.

The type of CPE induced by a virus is sometimes quite characteristic, so that an infecting agent can often be identified by the CPE it causes. In some cases the virus may increase the permeability of the plasma membrane so that the cytoplasm of the cell escapes and the plasma membrane collapses around the remaining nucleus; in other viral infections cells characteristically detach from a substratum, and in still others, the cell seems to burst open so that only debris survives the virus infection.

Cell damage is not the only response to virus infections. In fact, several viruses cause what might be considered the very opposite effect in that they stimulate cells to proliferate; often this is accompanied by a morphological transformation of the infected cells together with an altered growth pattern. In such cases, virus genetic information is sometimes integrated into the DNA of the cell.

Viruses that characteristically induce such changes in tissue cultures often cause tumors in animals; there are both RNA- and DNA-containing tumor viruses. The most important RNA tumor viruses insofar as studies with interferon are concerned are murine leukemia virus and mouse mammary tumor virus. Among the DNA tumor viruses, many studies have been performed on SV40.

Viral infections may also induce a number of changes in the plasma membranes of infected cells. These are usually as a result of insertion of virus proteins into the plasma membrane, a process that confers on the cell surface some of the properties of the newly inserted proteins. In some cases infected cells will agglutinate red blood cells, react with antibodies to viral antigens, or respond in a wholly new manner to various substances. Virus infections may also alter the plasma membrane by reorganizing its lipid constituents, but often these are not changed by infection.

A frequent outcome of virus infections is death of the cell; however, cells may survive and go on producing virus, a chronic infection. In some cases, chronic infections do not involve an obvious morphological change in cells, although viral antigens are induced on the cell surface. For instance, mouse cells can be chronically infected in culture with murine leukemia viruses. These agents cause leukemias in mice but usually induce only chronic infections in cultured mouse fibroblasts. Such chronically infected cells may continually produce very large quantities of virus without appearing to undergo any significant morphological alterations whatsoever.

Other chronic infections may show more viral effects. In some a large percentage of a culture may carry a latent infection with a virus that is ordinarily quite cytopathic. Characteristic of this type of infection is the chronic production of low titers of virus with traces of CPE when the culture is examined closely. Occasionally, for various reasons a chronically infected culture of this sort may destabilize, resulting in a rapid increase in virus titers and development of virus-induced CPE. Interferons may sometimes play a role in the development of such chronic virus infections.

THE ANTIVIRAL STATE

The mechanism of interferon action, for the sake of discussion, may be divided into two phases. The first relates to how interferon treatment induces an antiviral state or other activities in cells; the second, to how these induced states are expressed on various biological activities such as virus growth, cell replication, or the immune response.

Figure 10 is taken from a study in which AKR mouse cell monolayers were treated with 100 units of partially purified mouse interferon. The interferon was allowed to incubate with some of the cultures for 96 hr; in other cultures the interferon was washed off after 48 hr and the cultures were permitted to incubate for an additional 48 hr in medium. Several points are illustrated in this experiment and that in Fig. 2. Some antiviral activity develops within the first 2 hrs of incubation; in fact, the higher the concentration of interferon, the more rapidly the antiviral activity develops. In addition, the maximum antiviral activity that develops is dependent on concentration of interferon added.

The antiviral activity increased over a 16 hr period. It remained stable after reaching about a thousandfold inhibition of virus growth at that time and so long as the same concentration of interferon remained on the cells; however, if the interferon was washed off, the antiviral state decreased, so that no activity was observed 48 hr after washing.

The kinetics of the development and the disappearance of the antiviral state differ from cell type to cell type, in some cases being considerably faster than is seen in Fig. 10. There also appear to be a differences in the kinetics of development of antiviral activity after treatment with different types of interferon. Among human interferons, for instance, gamma interferon is reported to be slower than alpha or beta in inducing an antiviral state.

In any one cell type the degree of sensitivity of different viruses to interferons varies greatly; moreover, the order of sensitivity of different viruses changes with the cell type. For instance, arboviruses are very sensitive to interferon in chick cells,

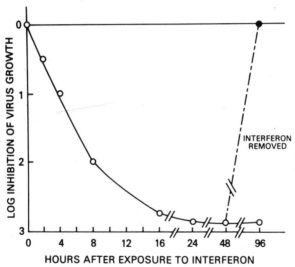

Fig. 10. Time course of development of antiviral activity following interferon treatment of mouse cells.

Mouse L cells were treated with 100 mouse interferon international reference units. At the time points indicated the interferon was removed and the cells were washed three times and then infected with EMC virus at a virus-to-cell multiplicity of 10:1. After 14 hr the culture fluids were harvested and assayed for virus. The results of the titration were expressed in terms of $\log_{10}$, subtracted from the titers in untreated controls, and expressed as the log inhibition of virus growth. After 48 hr of interferon treatment interferon was removed from one culture and the cells were permitted to incubate for an additional 48 hr before being infected with EMC virus (broken line marks interferon removed).

but in mouse cells vesicular stomatitis virus (VSV), a rhabdovirus, is more sensitive to interferon than is Sindbis virus, an arbovirus. In some species, such as the rabbit, DNA viruses are sometimes completely insensitive to interferon, and, indeed, infection with vaccinia virus or pseudorabies virus decreases the antiviral activity of interferon for RNA viruses. The reasons for these differences are not yet known, but they may be related to the multiple mechanisms of the antiviral action of interferons (discussed below) or differences in the replicative mechanisms of various viruses. The antiviral state against a given class of viruses could depend on a single mechanism of interferon action. If the action does not take place in a given cell type, the cells will be completely sensitive to that class of viruses in spite of treatment with high concentrations of interferon.

In order to bring about their effects on cells interferons must first react with the plasma membrane. The significant reaction is a binding of interferon, which is not an energy-requiring process. Under some conditions the bound interferon can be destroyed by trypsin with subsequent failure to develop an antiviral state. Later, bound interferon is spontaneously released from the cell surface without influencing the development of an antiviral state. Interferon may have a specific cell surface receptor; evidence for the specificity of the binding site is the finding that interferon action can be blocked in human cells by an antibody to a product of chromosome 21 or competitively by thryroid-stimulating hormone, chorionic gonadotropin, or cholera toxin. Since the latter three active biological substances appear to have specific binding sites that may be similar, it follows that interferon may bind to the same or to a very similar site as polypeptide substances do in this general group. There is some evidence that the species specificity of interferon action is not determined by its binding to a specific site, since mouse interferon may bind to cells in which it does not induce antiviral activity. Binding seems, therefore, necessary but not sufficient for the development of antiviral activity.

There is some information on the location and chemical nature of the putative interferon binding site. It appears to be on the outer surface of the plasma membrane. This was determined by stimulating human fibroblasts with polyIC to produce a type beta interferon in the presence of antibody to human beta interferon. Antiviral activity failed to develop in cells that were producing interferon; this meant that the interferon had to be externalized for it to induce an intracellular antiviral state. Other studies indicated that the chemical nature of the interferon receptor is a complex that contains both ganglioside and glycoprotein components. How these interact to bind interferon on the cell surface and transmit information to an intracellular site is not clear, since in *in vitro* experiments interferon binds to either the gangliosides or the glycoprotein. It is possible that the glycoprotein component represents an activation or amplification site for the induction of intracellular antiviral activity; similar mechanisms have been proposed for polypeptide hormone action.

Once interferon has interacted with its cell surface receptor, it is not clear what steps follow immediately. For instance, it is uncertain whether or not interferon is taken up by the cell. Some evidence indicates that it is not, because interferons bound to beads are active in inducing an antiviral state. It is not clear in such studies, however, how tightly the interferons are bound to the carrier. The activity of interferons can be accounted for by reactions initiated at the cell surface, but studies with purified, radioactive interferons will be necessary to answer definitively the question of whether interferon uptake is required for its biological activities. The great specific activity of interferons suggests that one or fewer molecules per cell can induce an antiviral state; it is therefore still possible that uptake does occur.

Cellular protein and RNA synthesis and possibly the elaboration of cyclic AMP are required for the development of the antiviral state after interferon treatment. The genetic locus for human interferon sensitivity is on the long arm of chromosome 21. This could code for an interferon receptor; it is also possible that it contains an operon for several functions related to interferon action or that these functions lie on the long arm of chromosome 21 in various loci. Indeed, sensitivity to interferon is related in human cells to the number of copies of chromosome 21 that are present; trisomic 21 cells (as in Down's syndrome) develop higher levels of antiviral activity than do diploid cells, which are in turn more sensitive than haploid cells. It will be important to determine exactly what chromosome 21 contributes to the development of antiviral activity to human interferon.

VIRUS REPLICATION IN INTERFERON-TREATED CELLS

Interferons inhibit the replication of a surprisingly wide variety of viruses, as well as some nonviral infectious agents, many of which have very little in common. A number of virologists have, therefore, investigated this problem and employed several virus-cell systems in attempts to find a specific virus function that is blocked in interferon-treated cells. At least four possible sites of action have been seriously suggested. The theories about interferon action currently in vogue are discussed in the order that they generally appear in the virus replication cycle.

Virus Uncoating

Until recently, there seemed little reason for seriously considering virus uncoating as a site of action for interferons. Several studies with infectious viral RNAs indicated from positive-stranded viruses that interferons inhibited their replication. These data suggested that interferon acts at a site beyond the uncoating step.

One study with simian virus 40 (SV40) seemed, however, to contradict the findings with infectious RNA. The production of SV40 early mRNA and T antigen was markedly inhibited in interferon-treated monkey cells, when these cells were infected with intact SV40. If, however, infectious SV40 deoxyribonucleic acid (DNA) was employed, the results were directly opposite to those obtained with infectious RNA. The synthesis of early SV40 mRNA and T antigen was only slightly inhibited in interferon-treated cells infected with the SV40 DNA. This would appear to indicate that in interferon-treated cells, SV40 uncoating, or a step soon after it, was inhibited and that this is the explanation for the apparent inhibition of SV40-directed transcription under these conditions. A similar block in uncoating or an event soon thereafter has been described at nonpermissive conditions for an SV40 mutant.

These results in interferon-treated cells infected with SV40 DNA seemed clear-cut, but additional studies have provided directly contradictory results, so that it is not at present possible to say definitively whether virus uncoating is altered in interferon-treated cells.

Virus Transcription

Work on interferon inhibition of transcription is quite controversial. The disagreement revolves around whether interferon treatment causes an inhibition in the primary transcription of the genetic information of viruses. All the possible answers can be found in various publications.

Part of the confusion undoubtedly is due to the close relationship between viral RNA synthesis and viral protein synthesis. If a virus requires a polymerase not present in cells and has no endogenous RNA polymerase as a structural element, inhibition of viral protein synthesis will result in inhibition of all virus-directed RNA synthesis, because the viral polymerase is among the proteins whose synthesis would be inhibited. Arboviruses and picornaviruses, among the RNA positive-stranded viruses commonly used in interferon research, are lacking structural polymerases.

In the case of those agents containing structural polymerases, negative-stranded viruses, analysis of the site of inhibition can be quite complicated. Since a polymerase is already present, inhibition of protein synthesis does not cause inhibition of early RNA synthesis. Primary transcription takes place in these cells, but secondary transcription, which depends on the elaboration of new polymerases, will be inhibited. Results obtained employing such systems require careful analysis, since significant inhibition of RNA synthesis does not necessarily indicate that primary RNA synthesis is the site of action.

Among RNA viruses, there have been detailed reports on the effect of interferon on the primary transcription of vesicular stomatitis virus (VSV), influenza virus, and reovirus. In the case of DNA viruses, vaccinia virus and SV40 have been well studied.

Inhibition of primary transcription of VSV has been reported in human, chick, and monkey cells. These studies employed cycloheximide to block secondary transcription and actinomycin D to inhibit most RNA synthesis; the viral RNA synthesis was then measured in the presence or absence of interferon. In the experiments performed in human cells, there was a quantitative decrease in viral mRNA but no qualitative change.

These results certainly suggested that at least one effect of interferon was to inhibit primary transcription of RNA viruses with structural polymerases. Contradictory results have, however, been obtained in a study of interferon inhibition of VSV replication in interferon-treated monkey or human cells. With concentrations of interferon that significantly inhibited virus replication in these systems, there was only a 30% decrease in the specific activity of viral RNA synthesis in the presence of cycloheximide and interferon in monkey cells as compared with those treated with cycloheximide alone. In the human cells, the comparable figure was 53%. Those viral RNA forms that were most sensitive to inhibition by interferons were forms that required the elaboration of a new polymerase to produce and so were due to secondary transcription. In addition, a concentration of interferon that inhibited viral RNA synthesis by only 10% inhibited viral protein synthesis by 60%. A study of the effect of interferon on early production of viral RNA in VSV or influenza virus-infected chick or mouse cells also reached the conclusion that inhibition of primary transcription was probably not the basis of interferon action.

In study on the mechanism of inhibition of reovirus replication by interferon, the authors employed a different tack. Among the temperature-sensitive mutants of reovirus type 3, one is blocked in its formation of progeny RNA at nonpermissive temperatures (38.5°C); therefore, only primary transcription takes place at this temperature. A study of the growth of this mutant in interferon-treated cells incubated at 38.5°C indicated that a concentration of interferon that inhibited virus yields by 80%, inhibited primary transcription by only 12%. Under approximately the same conditions, however, virus-directed translations was significantly inhibited (see the following discussion).

One additional finding in interferon-treated cells infected with an RNA virus will be discussed, although strictly speaking it does not deal with an inhibition of transcription. Treatment with chick interferon caused an elevation of the enzymatic activity of a membrane-associated RNase with optimal activity at an alkaline pH (assays were run at pH 8). If this is a general finding, it could explain some of the divergent observations that have been made on interferon action in various laboratories. It would, for instance, account for why viral transcription seems to be inhibited in some interferon-treated cells, whereas in others, viral translation seems to be the site of interferon action. By this theory, what results one obtains would depend on what was being measured. Intracellular viral mRNA concentrations would be decreased and virus-directed translation would be inhibited. In cell-free systems measuring viral translation, the increased nuclease in extracts of interferon-treated cells might hydrolyze the added viral mRNA, and this in turn would cause an apparent primary inhibition in translation.

In order for these notions to be considered as a general mechanism of interferon action, however, it would have to be shown that increased alkaline RNase was induced by homologous interferons in cells of species other than chicks and only chick cells were used; indeed, others have reported no increase in nuclease activity in polyIC-treated monkey, hamster, quail, or duck cell extracts. In addition, no specificity was shown by this system, in that the RNase activity was tested only with VSV mRNA. Since interferon action appears to show specificity for virus functions, an RNase that is thought to be responsible for interferon action might show a restricted spectrum of activity.

Vaccinia virus was the first of the DNA viruses to be studied intensively with respect to interferons. In many ways vaccinia virus infection lends itself well to this sort of study, because the virus contains an RNA polymerase that is activated with removal of the outer coat in the virus. The polymerase, which is located in the viral core, then elaborates viral mRNA, which is translated to yield several active proteins, including one that inhibits activity of the virus structural RNA polymerase and another that is responsible for final uncoating of the viral DNA.

The effects of interferon on this well-studied system are fairly clear-cut. Early vaccinia mRNA synthesis was increased, but final uncoating of the viral DNA was inhibited. Although the production of viral mRNA depends on a virus-associated polymerase, the inhibition of the activity of the polymerase and the uncoating of the viral DNA depend on synthesis of new proteins. It would appear in this system, then, that the site of interferon-induced antiviral action must lie between virus-directed transcription and translation.

SV40 differs from the other DNA viruses discussed in that it lacks a structural RNA polymerase and so at least early in infection must depend on a cellular polymerase. Interferon treatment inhibited SV40 T antigen production in acutely infected but not in transformed cells (see the following discussion). Transformation of mouse 3T3 cells by SV40 was also inhibited by interferon treatment. These results were consistent with a primary effect on either virus uncoating or virus-directed transcription or translation.

The effect of interferon treatment on early SV40-specific RNA synthesis in monkey cells was also studied. The results indicated a marked inhibition of very early RNA synthesis under conditions where no late RNA could be formed, that is, in cells treated with enough cytosine arabinoside to inhibit viral DNA synthesis by more than 99%. A subsequent study showed that the inhibition of early SV40 RNA synthesis in interferon-treated cells was probably not the result of inhibition of virus adsorption, penetration, or uncoating; of increased degradation of either the viral DNA template or viral RNA; or, finally, of an inhibition of translation of a very early mRNA that might have a secondary inhibitory effect on further early viral RNA synthesis. These results with SV40 were somewhat unexpected, because the virus must use a cell polymerase early in infection.

One other study with the SV40 system is of present interest. SV40 RNA prepared *in vitro* with SV40 DNA and a bacterial polymerase was microinjected into SV40-permissive monkey cells that had been treated with interferon. Under these conditions, T antigen production was blocked, although it was evident in controls microinjected but not treated with interferon. This result indicted that, in interferon-treated and SV40-infected cells, translation of virus genetic information may be inhibited; however, this result does not necessarily mean that inhibition of translation is an important mechanism of interferon action in the SV40 system *in vivo*.

Although many studies reviewed in this section suggested that interferon treatment caused an inhibition in early virus-directed transcription, in the case of most virus groups there is at least one study that indicated no direct effect of interferon treatment on primary transcription. With RNA viruses having virus-associated polymerases, the most meaningful studies of interferon action at this point would appear to be those that employ viral mutants blocked just after primary transcription has been completed. The general conclusions reached by such studies was that, although there was some inhibitory effect of interferon treatment on early RNA synthesis, it was not enough to account for the profound inhibition of virus replication.

As for DNA viruses, the weight of the evidence in the case of vaccinia virus infection is that interferon treatment has no inhibitory effect on primary viral RNA synthesis. On the other hand, early mRNA synthesis directed by SV40 does appear to be inhibited under some conditions.

Viral Protein Synthesis

Before discussing evidence that interferon treatment inhibits viral protein synthesis, it should be noted again that viral protein and RNA synthesis are so interdependent that it is often difficult to distinguish which of the two is the primary site of action of an antiviral substance such as interferon, since progeny RNA molecules are usually responsible for most of the total virus-directed protein and RNA synthesis that is carried on during infection. Therefore, whether interferon treatment acts directly to inhibit RNA or protein synthesis early in infection, later both transcription and translation are profoundly inhibited. In order to show which of the two is the primary site of interferon action, it is necessary to study its effect under conditions in which viral RNA and protein synthesis are clearly dissociated. This has been effected in two ways: The first involves studying viral protein synthesis in cell-free systems. The second involves studying, in infected cells, the messenger function of parental (input) RNA of viruses (the genome of which is an mRNA, i.e., positive-stranded RNA viruses) or the messenger function of the viral mRNA that is made by using the input RNA as a template in association with a viral polymerase (negative-stranded RNA viruses). There have also been important studies on one DNA virus. Experiments on viral mRNA function in cell-free systems derived from interferon-treated cells will also be discussed.

Semliki Forest virus (SFV, an arbovirus) and mengovirus (a picornavirus) have been used to determine whether positive-stranded RNA virus messenger function is a primary site of interferon action. Of the negative-stranded RNA viruses, VSV and reovirus protein synthesis have been employed. Among the DNA viruses there has been extensive study of the effect of interferon treatment only on the early protein synthesis of vaccinia virus.

In infection with SFV, inhibition of viral protein synthesis in interferon-treated cells does not appear to be a result of inhibition of viral RNA synthesis. Under conditions in which viral RNA synthesis was almost completely inhibited, early SFV protein synthesis was unaffected. If cells were treated with interferon, however, no virus-specific proteins could be identified. In this system, therefore, parental RNA does not seem to be translated.

Only one study has been carried out on the effect of interferon treatment on protein synthesis directed by the negative-stranded RNA virus VSV. The results indicated that 3 hr after infection in interferon-treated rabbit kidney cells, the formation of all structural and nonstructural VSV proteins was inhibited. Viral RNA synthesis was not studied, but the inhibition of viral protein synthesis was so profound that, if decreased RNA synthesis were the primary factor, only a very marked inhibition could possibly account for these results. The findings in interferon-treated, VSV-infected cells indicated that, even if it does occur, inhibition of virus-directed primary transcription might not be as great as would be necessary to account completely for the observed inhibition of virus-directed protein synthesis.

In the study of the effect of interferon on the growth of a reovirus mutant, the results of which were discussed earlier with respect to primary viral transcription, inhibition of viral protein synthesis was also studied. Under conditions in which only primary transcription took place, there was a 20% inhibition in viral RNA synthesis but a 40–72% inhibition of the synthesis of various individual virus-specific polypeptides. The apparent inhibition of viral RNA synthesis did not seem great enough to account for all the observed inhibition of virus translation.

In interferon-treated cells infected with vaccinia virus, as indicated earlier, several studies indicated that early viral mRNA synthesis was not inhibited. The vaccinia virus mRNA formed in interferon-treated cells has a normal content of polyadenylic acid, but it does not associate with ribosomes to form polyribosomes as readily as does mRNA ordinarily formed early in vaccinia virus infections. This failure to form polyribosomes readily is probably the result of an inhibition of the initiation steps in viral protein synthesis, although some inhibition of chain elongation was also reported. There was a suggestion that the site of inhibition of initiation of peptide synthesis might be in the formation of a complex between a vaccinia virus mRNA-protein (ribonucleoprotein) and a ribosomal subunit; however, the findings did not show this conclusively.

SV40 is the only other DNA virus in which virus-directed protein synthesis in interferon-treated cells has been studied to any extent. In interferon-treated cells there is marked inhibition of the synthesis of viral T antigen in lytic infections. As previously noted, there was inhibition of the translation of SV40 mRNA microinjected into interferon-treated cells. This suggests that translation might take place in interferon-treated cells; however, significant inhibition of virus uncoating or transcription would preclude there being very much SV40 mRNA produced in interferon-treated cells. When interferon was added later in infection with SV40, however, the results were somewhat unexpected. The uncoating of SV40 and the production of SV40-mRNA were not inhibited under these conditions, but production of virus-specific proteins was decreased. The very significant differences obtained in studies adding interferon before or late in SV40 infection re-

63

main unexplained. They indicate that the effects of interferon can be multifocal even with infection by a single virus.

In the study of interferon's effect on virus-directed protein synthesis, two sorts of cell-free systems have been employed. In the earlier group of experiments, viral RNA was incubated with extracts from control or interferon-treated cells, and the interactions were analyzed with respect to the binding of the RNA to the cellular components. Later, when cell-free systems employing components from animal cells became available for the production of specific polypeptides, several laboratories began to study the ability of viral RNA to stimulate amino acid incorporation by cytoplasmic fractions from interferon-treated and control cells.

The results of studies on the first type of system were inconclusive. There were some reports that in cells treated with interferon, binding of viral mRNA to ribosomes was inhibited; in other studies ribosomes from interferon-treated cells bound viral mRNA as well as did control ribosomes.

Although the nature of the RNA and protein synthesis required for interferon action is still uncertain, the recent development of some understanding of the activities of interferon-induced enzymes in cell-free systems is one of the most important aspects of studies on interferon. As noted earlier, it has been recognized for several years that in cultures of interferon-treated, virus-infected cells, viral messenger RNA was not efficiently translated. In some cases where virion-associated transcriptases were present, interferon treatment did not inhibit viral messenger RNA synthesis. In cell-free protein-synthesizing systems derived from mouse cells treated with low but still highly effective concentrations of interferon, there was very little inhibition of viral messenger RNA translation unless the cells from which the extracts were derived had also been infected with a virus after interferon treatment. This suggested that interferon treatment induced a potential antiviral state that was not fully developed until the cells had been virus infected. In considering what factors might be involved in the activation of the antiviral state in extracts from interferon-treated cells, it was found that addition of minute quantities of double-stranded RNA to extracts of interferon-treated, but not untreated, control cells resulted in the inhibition of viral protein synthesis. This might be related to the requirement for viral infection of interferon-treated cells in order to demonstrate an inhibition of translation of viral messenger RNA, because in many viral infections double-stranded RNA species are produced.

Treatment of cell extracts from interferon-treated cells with double-stranded RNA induces the production of at least three substances that appear related to antiviral activity (Fig. 11). These are a protein kinase, a series of oligoadenylate polymers with a 2', 5' linkage, the most important of which is the trimer, $pppA2'p5'A2'p5'A_{OH}$ (2', 5'A for short), and a synthetase that catalyzes the production of the oligo-A polymers. The protein kinase is induced by interferon and activated by double-stranded RNA in extracts from interferon-treated cells; this kinase phosphorylates the small subunit of the protein synthesis initiation factor eIF-2, an action consistent with several observations strongly suggesting that initiation of viral protein synthesis was inhibited following interferon treatment. In order for the kinase to be activated, it itself must be phosphorylated. There is also present in cells a phosphatase activity that can readily dephosphorylate the kinase, but it appears that effective activators of the kinase, such as polyIC, also inhibit the phosphatase (Fig. 11).

The 2',5'A, on the other hand, is synthesized from ATP by another interferon-induced enzyme, adenylate synthetase, which is also activated by double-stranded RNA; 2',5'A can be destroyed by a phosphodiesterase or degradase present in cells. The 2',5'A that is produced by the synthetase inhibits protein synthesis by activating an endoribonuclease present in cells. This enzyme hydrolyzes messenger RNA so that elongation of nascent chains of viral proteins is inhibited. Thus there are at least two general ways in which interferon treatment inhibits virus-directed protein synthesis (Fig. 11), but it is uncertain which, if either, of these is the more significant in a given virus infection of interferon-treated cells. Both may contribute to an antiviral state, although precisely how is at present unclear, since it has not yet been shown that these mechanisms of protein synthesis inhibition are specific for virus-directed functions. Rather than being unique antiviral mechanisms, the processes employed in the interferon system may well be adaptations of the normal systems that con-

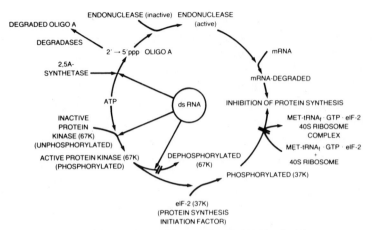

Fig. 11. Double-stranded ribonucleic acid (dsRNA)-related steps in the mechanism of interferon action.

In the case of the kinase, in the presence of dsRNA and adenosine triphosphate (ATP), an active protein kinase with a molecular weight of 67,000 (67K) is formed. The phosphate added to the kinase may be removed by a phosphatase that is inhibited in the presence of dsRNA. The function of the active protein kinase appears to be to add a phosphate group to a subunit with an molecular weight of 37,000 (37K) of protein synthesis initiation factor eIF-2. The phosphorylated 37K is not active when it is added to the initiation factor eIF-2. Ordinarily, eIF-2 acts together with a ribosomal subunit (40S), initiator transfer RNA (Met-tRNA$_f$), and guanosine triphosphate (GTP) to initiate protein synthesis. In the presence of the phosphosylated 37K subunit of eIF-2, the initiation of protein synthesis is inhibited. In the case of the 2′,5′-A synthetase, the addition of dsRNA activated the enzyme which forms oligoadenylate polymers (2′,5′ ppp oligo A) from ATP. Several degradases may inactivate oligo A, but, if it is not destroyed, the oligo A interacts with an endonuclease that is present in most cells. The active endonuclease degrades messenger RNA (mRNA). This in turn inhibits protein synthesis by stopping the elongation of proteins. Thus, both of these pathways may converge to inhibit viral protein synthesis.

trol cell growth and differentiation. It was not entirely unexpected, therefore, to find that interferons also have effects on the immune systems and on the growth of uninfected cells (Chapter 6).

Other studies have reported that interferon-treated cells were deficient in some species of tRNA. This might be an important mechanism of interferon action, if viral protein synthesis employed species of tRNA that were not important in cell metabolism. The results of these findings were, however, inconclusive in establishing whether the interferon effects on tRNA really contributed to the inhibition of virus replication.

Another interesting finding was the discovery of an inhibition of the addition of methyl groups to viral mRNA in extracts of interferon-treated cells. Most viral and cellular mRNAs contain blocked and methylated termini. This methyl group addition was necessary for the translation of some viral mRNAs in animal cell extracts. The methylation of unmethylated viral mRNA was significantly impaired in extracts from interferon-treated cells, but it is uncertain what the significance of these findings is, because interferon treatment also significantly inhibits the replication of viruses such as EMC that do not have methylated termini.

Terminal Steps in the Virus Replication Cycle

The effect of interferon treatment on RNA tumor virus replication differs from the already discussed mechanisms (Table XIII; Fig. 12). It has been known for many years that interferon treatment inhibited yields of murine leukemia viruses (MLV), but recent studies indicated that the synthesis of at least some (and possibly all) the virus-specific proteins of MLV was not inhibited in interferon-treated cells. Early steps in Friend virus maturation were inhibited in interferon-treated cells. The final stages in virus

TABLE XIII. Actions of Interferon on Membrane-Containing Viruses[a]

Class of inhibition	Level of inhibition	Examples of this type of inhibition
I.	Increase in intracisternal viral particles (which may be precursors of mature viral particles)	Friend leukemia virus-infected cells
II.	Virus particles stick to membrane of cell	AKR–MLV in AKR mouse cells; MMTV-infected cells.
III.	Virus particles produced with low infectivity	Moloney MLV in TB mouse cells; AKR–MLV in AKR cells; VSV in Ly cells

[a] Abbreviations: MLV, murine leukemia virus; VSV, vesicular stomatitis virus; MMTV, mouse mammary tumor virus.

67

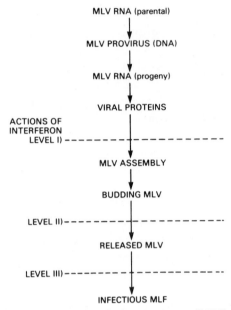

MLV RNA (parental)

MLV PROVIRUS (DNA)

MLV RNA (progeny)

VIRAL PROTEINS

ACTIONS OF
INTERFERON
LEVEL I) ------------+------------

MLV ASSEMBLY

BUDDING MLV

LEVEL II) ---------+---------

RELEASED MLV

LEVEL III) ---------+---------

INFECTIOUS MLF

Fig. 12. Interferon action on murine leukemia viruses (MLV).
Cells are infected with parental MLV. The MLV reverse transcriptase forms a proviral double-stranded, complementary DNA (cDNA) that serves as a template for making progeny MLV RNA. Some of this RNA serves the function of a messenger RNA (mRNA) that is translated to form MLV structural and functional proteins. The MLV RNA and proteins are assembled at the plasma membrane and the new virus buds from the cell surface. The virus formed includes a portion of the cell membrane that has been modified by insertion of viral proteins. The budding virus is released from the cell surface and undergoes further modification and maturation to form infectious MLV. Virus replication is inhibited on at least three levels in this process. In some systems, the assembly of virus proteins and RNA into particles seems to be inhibited (level I). In others, the ability of virus particles to bud from the cell surface is impaired, so that the plasma membrane of interferon-treated cells is covered with large numbers of particles whose budding has been slowed or aborted (level II). In still other systems, MLV is released from the cell but the particles formed are very low in infectivity. This is probably due to an abnormality in the viral glycoprotein (level III).

maturation were also the site of inhibition in AKR cells infected with MLV and in mouse cells chronically infected with mammary tumor virus (MMTV); therefore, virus was not efficiently released from the plasma membrane of the cell in these cases. In scanning electronmicrographs of the surface of interferon-treated, MMTV- or MLV-producing cells apparently morphologically normal virus particles were attached to the cell surface in much higher concentrations than were normally present. In other systems MLV morphogenesis and release were normal, but the MLV released from interferon-treated cells was markedly defective in infectivity.

The finding of a low infectivity-to-particle ratio was not, however, limited to MLV. In vesicular stomatitis virus (VSV)-infected mouse cells treated with low concentrations of interferon (3–30 IU/ml) a defective form of VSV was produced. This virus was deficient in glycoprotein (G protein); probably because of this, the virus morphologically lacked spikes on the outer surface of its membrane. Since these glycoprotein spikes represent viral attachment points vital for virus adsorption, the virus particles without them were noninfectious. Interestingly, the major abnormality in the noninfectious particles of both MLV and VSV produced by interferon-treated cells was a deficiency in the amount of their respective glycoproteins. The deficiency in glycosylation may be related to a decreased activity induced by low concentrations of interferon of a cell membrane associated transferase that initiates a series of reactions ending in the glycosylation of asparagine residues in peptides. The poorly glycosylated viral glycoproteins may be unstable in interferon-treated cells; this might lead to a serious shortage of this structural element at the time of virus assembly.

Therefore, what interferon treatment seems to do is to affect virus replication at several levels. There appear to be at least some instances of inhibition of virus-directed transcription, and inhibition of virus-directed protein synthesis takes place at several sites, including initiation and elongation of virus peptide formation (Fig. 11). If inhibition of virus-directed transcription or translation is not operative, membrane-associated viruses have yet another interferon-induced barrier to hurdle—the effects of interferon on their assembly. These latter effects are summarized in Table XIII; some may be due to inhibition of glycosylation of viral proteins. It is no wonder in view of these findings that the replication of such a wide spectrum of viruses is sensitive to interferon treatment. These facts may also explain why some virus might not be affected in interferon-treated cells in which the growth of other viruses is inhibited; this might be related to one or more mechanisms of antiviral action not being activated in the same interferon-treated cells in which other mechanisms are fully active.

RESTRICTIONS OF INTERFERON ACTION

There is a restriction of the antiviral action of interferons in virus-directed translation in systems in which the viral genome is integrated into an interferon-resistant virus or into a host genome. As noted earlier, interferon treatment also does not inhibit virus protein synthesis in cells producing murine leukemia virus (MLV). In view of what will be discussed, it is important to note that the messenger RNA of MLV is generated from a provirus integrated into the genome of the host.

In interferon-treated cells lytically infected with SV40 virus, not only was infectious virion formation inhibited but production of viral T antigen, an early gene product, was decreased, as was viral-induced cell transformation. The stimulation of cellular DNA synthesis in BHK-21 hamster cells after infection with polyoma virus (which is closely related to SV40) was also inhibited by treatment with hamster interferon. All of these findings clearly indicated that early SV40 and polyoma virus functions are sensitive to interferon treatment.

It was therefore surprising that in SV40 virus-transformed mouse cells the production of SV40 T antigen was insensitive to interferon treatment, in spite of the fact that such treatment made them resistant to VSV infection. That is, the same interferon system that recognized and inhibited new lytic infections with SV40 and other viruses such as VSV apparently failed to inhibit viral function, when it was exercised by an integrated tumor virus genome. This interpretation was strengthened by findings in cells infected with an adeno-SV40 hybrid virus that is infectious and presents an interesting covalent linkage of an interferon-sensitive (SV40 virus) with an interferon-insensitive (adenovirus) genome. In simultaneous infection of cells with both SV40 and adenovirus the sensitivity of adenovirus or SV40 T antigen production was characteristic of infection with either virus alone; however, in infection with the SV40-adenovirus hybrid, production of both T antigens was as resistant as adenovirus T antigen production in infection with adenovirus alone.

There is some independent evidence that the SV40 genome is covalently linked to the adenovirus genome in the hybrid or to cellular DNA in SV40-transformed cells. The messenger RNA produced by the integrated SV40 genome may contain host sequences, and the messenger RNA of the hybrid contains both adenovirus and SV40 sequences. The resistance of SV40 T antigen production to interferon treatment in the case of integrated genomes seems to indicate that the primary sequence of nucleotides in the genome does not determine sensitivity to interferons. Other sites on the genome, such as leader sequences concerned with initiation or control of genetic expression, would then be the loci of interferon action, since the presence of host- or interferon-resistant virus RNA sequences appears to render a virus messenger RNA resistant to interferon action. This interpretation is consistent with mechanisms of interferon action involving phosphorylation of protein synthesis initiation factor eIF-2 or hydrolysis of viral messenger RNA by an endonuclease. The specificity of such reactions (if they are indeed specific) may involve such unique sites on the viral genomes.

BIBLIOGRAPHY

Friedman, R. M. (1977). Antiviral activity of interferons. *Bact. Rev.* **41**, 543–567.
Revel, M. (1979). Molecular mechanisms involved in the antiviral effects of interferon. *Interferon* **1**, 101–163.

6
OTHER ACTIONS OF INTERFERONS

Studies reporting that interferons had activities other than their antiviral effects date back to 1958, the year after interferons were discovered. For a long period the interpretation of results on studies of nonantiviral actions of interferons were clouded by the knowledge that only a small percentage of the material in the preparations employed was actually interferon. The recent availability of purified preparations of interferons has brought an end to doubts about whether these effects were indeed due to interferon itself or to contaminants of interferon preparations. Since most of the reported actions can now be demonstrated to be associated with the purified preparations available, it is quite respectable to write a chapter on nonantiviral effects of interferons.

One nonantiviral effect of interferons that has been studied extensively for many years has already been discussed; it is the priming interferon production by interferon treatment. This was originally regarded as resulting from inhibition of viral cytopathic activity; that is, the pretreatment with interferon prevented or delayed the cell damage induced by virus infection. This in turn permitted the induction of larger amounts of interferon. This theory cannot account, however, for priming following induction by polyIC. Therefore, this nonantiviral effect of interferon treatment is probably related to an action on interferon messenger RNA production, rather than on cell protection.

EFFECTS ON THE IMMUNE SYSTEM

Interferons have profound effects on many different immunlogical reactions. They may inhibit some reactions while enhancing others. All the effector cells of the immune system may be influenced by interferon treatment and the effects may be expressed in *in vitro* as well as *in vivo* systems (Table XIV).

In order to understand the effects of interferons on the immune system, it is necessary to review the functions of some of the types of cells that play a part in the immune response. Thymus-derived (T) lymphocytes are cells that originate in bone marrow but migrate and settle in the thymus. In this location they mature and gain their functional capacities, which are directed at many cellular immune responses. When T lymphocytes come in contact

TABLE XIV. Effects of Interferons on Various Aspects of the Immune System

Effector cell	Function and effect of interferons	
	In vitro	*In vivo*
B	Antibody formation early treatment—decreased late treatment—increased	Antibody formation early—decreased late—increased
T(cell-mediated immunity)	Mixed lymphocyte reaction-decreased H-2 antigen expression—increased Mitogenic response—increased	Graft versus host reaction—decreased H-2 antigen expression—increased Delayed-type hypersensitivity (sensitization and response)—decreased Allograft rejection—delayed
Non-B, Non-T	Killer or natural killer activity—increased	Killer or natural killer activity—increased
Macrophage (nonspecific resistance)	Phagocytosis—increased Antitumor cell activity—increased	Phagocytosis—increased Antitumor cell activity—increased

with an antigen for which they have specific receptors, they divide to produce additional T lymphocytes with the same specificity. They also change in character and acquire the ability (1) to produce various active biological substances called lymphokines that can attract or activate components of the immune system, or act directly as immunomodulators (gamma interferon itself is a lymphokine), and (2) to act as helper or suppressor cells that can modulate the activities of the other major group of lymphocytes (B lymphocytes).

B lymphocytes also originate in bone marrow, but they mature in sites other than the thymus. When a mature B lymphocyte comes in contact with an antigen for which it has specific receptors, it is stimulated to divide and to differentiate into a plasma cell. Plasma cells are antibody-producing factories that make antibodies with the same specificity as the receptors on the B lymphocyte from which they are derived. B lymphocytes interact with helper T lymphocytes that may increase (helper function) or decrease (suppressor function) the antibody-producing capacity of B cells.

Some other types of lymphocytes with important functions are neither T nor B cells. Natural killer cells (NK cells) comprise one group of these. NK cells are non-B, non-T lymphocytes that can interact with antigens on a cell surface and thus bring about the lysis of that cell; usually NK cells affect the cytolysis of either virus-infected or tumor cells. Another non-T, non-B lymphocyte is the killer cell that also affects cytolysis, but, unlike the NK cell, requires specific antibody to carry out this process. This is therefore an antibody-dependent lymphocyte cytotoxicity.

One other cell type that is important in the immune response and is regulated by interferons is the macrophage. Macrophages are a diverse group of cells, excluding granulocytes, which have the capacity to engulf and destroy foreign material.

Interferon treatment has varied affects on antibody-forming B cells. The primary or the secondary antibody response can be inhibited or enhanced; the particular effect depends on the concentration of interferon employed and whether the exposure of the B cells to interferon is before or after antigen sensitization. Interferon treatment of B cells in both *in vivo* and *in vitro* systems before exposure to antigens resulted in very significant inhibition of antibody production. The primary and secondary responses to a thymus-dependent antigen (sheep red blood cells, SBRC) or to a thymus-independent antigen (lypopolysaacharide) were inhibited. This may have been due to an inhibition in the number of proliferating clones; thus, it may be related to the growth-inhibiting properties of interferon. In addition, treatment with interferon before sensitization with antigen also inhibited the function of memory cells in the immune system. When mice were exposed to interferon before immunization with SRBC, there was a marked suppressive effect on secondary responses of SRBC even very long after primary interferon treatment.

Administration of interferon after sensitization with antigen resulted in an altogether different effect, however. With interferon treatment of animals or of lymphocyte cultures 3–4 days after antigenic stimulation there was significant enhancement of the immune response. This appeared to be due to an effect of interferon on immune cell proliferation or function; in this case the effect may have been on suppressor T cells that modulate the immune response, so that, although late addition of interferon did not seriously affect the functions of B cells, T cells that appear to moderate the amplitude of the immune response were apparently inhibited. This resulted in production of larger quantities of antibody than were made in the absence of interferon.

The response of B cells was also dose dependent. Very low concentrations of interferon caused enhancement of antibody production, whereas high concentrations resulted in its inhibition. It is of interest to note the similarity between this observation and interferon priming and blocking, since low or moderate concentrations of interferon often enhance interferon production, whereas high concentrations result in decreased production.

The type of interferon used to influence antibody production was important. On the basis of antiviral activity, gamma interferon was 250 times more effective on the immune mechanism than alpha or beta interferons; however, such differences between gamma interferon, on the one hand, and alpha or beta interferons, on the other, may not signify that gamma interferon is necessarily a specific modulator for the immune system, since the specific antiviral activity of gamma interferon is still unknown and could be significantly lower than that of the other human interferons. Therefore, on a molar basis the activity of the interferons may not differ in the immune system, since the antiviral activity of gamma interferon could be 250 times less than alpha or beta interferons.

Interferons can also affect the IgE system; treatment of mouse spleen cells with interferon resulted in a decreased ability to transfer cutaneous anaphylaxis. In addition, interferon treatment increased the release of histamine from basophils after exposure to ragweed antigen or to anti-IgE antibody; therefore, production of interferon may play a role in the frequent development of allergic symptoms such as asthmatic attacks during viral respiratory infections.

Interferon treatment altered many T-cell-mediated immune mechanisms. *In vitro* studies indicated that pretreatment with interferon inhibited cell proliferation in the mixed lymphocyte response. Interferon also increased the expression of H-2^d and H-2^k transplantation antigens on mouse spleen cells, splenic T lymphocytes, and thymic lymphocytes. This observation may be related to the finding that interferon enhanced the expression of tumor antigens on the surface of tumor cells. Thus, interferon concomitantly had effects on both cell differentiation and cell proliferation.

In *in vivo* studies in the mouse, interferon treatment also affected many aspects of cell-mediated immunity. In the graft-versus-host reaction both cell proliferation and murine leukemia virus activation were inhibited by interferon treatment. Other cell-mediated immune responses were altered by interferon treatment: allograft rejection was delayed in mice receiving exogenous interferon, and in the delayed hypersensitivity response, interferon treatment inhibited both the sensitization to antigen and the tissue response to a test antigen.

In non-T, non-B lymphocytes interferon treatment increased the cell-killing activity of NK and of killer cells. In contrast to most of the reports of inhibitory effects of interferon treatment on antibody production and cell-mediated immunity, interferon treatment apparently stimulated almost all the macrophage functions that have been studied. The results of these reports suggested that interferon is a monocyte- or macrophage-activating factor. *In vivo* and *in vitro* phagocytosis by macrophages was increased by interferon treatment; this appeared to be due both to an increase in the number of particles taken up per cell and to an increase in the percentage of cells engaged in phagocytosis. Although interferon treatment inhibited the maturation of monocytes into macrophages, it enhanced the tumor cells growth-inhibiting properties of resting mouse peritoneal macrophages. Interfons are, however, difficult to separate from macrophage-activating factors, so it is not clear that these effects are exclusively due to interferon and not to a contaminant in the interferon preparation. It is important to consider this as a general *caveat*, since many lymphokines may be difficult to separate from interferons. This is especially true when considering work on gamma interferons, because the methods used to stimulate their production (with mitogens or antigens) also induce the synthesis of lymphokine activities. Therefore, although a healthy skepticism about reports of interferons on the immune system is in order, at least until the nature of lymphokines is better elucidated, interferons certainly appear to be important regulatory factors in many aspects of the immune response. Some of these activities may be related to the general growth inhibitory properties of interferon, but others seem to be especially adapted to regulation for the immune system. It is possible that gamma interferons are specific regulatory substances for the immune system; additional research on gamma interferons should aid in establishing their significance.

EFFECTS ON CELL GROWTH AND DIFFERENTIATION

The inhibition of cell growth that is caused by treatment with interferons should by differentiated from toxic effects interferons may induce. The former is a slowing of cell growth with no cytopathic effect; the latter is due to cell damage induced by interferons in conjunction with another factor. This additional factor may be a virus or another substance. For instance, cytopathic damage induced by double-stranded RNA, or vaccinia, influenza, or vesicular stomatitis viruses is more rapid and severe in interferon-treated than in control cells. In addition, some interferon-treated cells are very sensitive to the toxic effect of double-stranded RNA forms.

On the other hand, interferons have been reported to slow the growth rate of many normal and transformed cells. Even some intracellular microorganisms are sensitive to the growth inhibitory effects of interferons. These organisms include *S. flexneri* among bacteria; *R. akai*, a rickettsia; the Chlamydiae *C. psittacosis* and *C. trachomatis*; and, among protozoa, the intracellular growth stages of *P. berghei* and *T. gondii*.

The inhibitory effect of interferons on animal cell growth is reversible; it involves a slowing of growth observable in both cell cultures and *in vivo*. In fact, one toxic action of interferons in clinical studies is on bone marrow, ordinarily a rapidly replicating tissue. In newborn mice, interferon treatment causes a wasting leading to death due to hepatic toxicity, whereas, in human newborns treated for congenital cytomegalovirus infection with large doses of interferon, failure to thrive was observed so that interferon treatment had to be suspended (noted in Chapter 8).

Substances such as interferons that inhibit cell growth are often especially effective inhibitors of the proliferation of the most rapidly growing cells, tumors. Several hypotheses have been advanced to explain the antitumor activity of interferons (Table XV). The last three have already been discussed in this chapter. Let it suffice to mention again that they may legitimately be listed as antitumor mechanisms.

The antitumor activity of interferons could be simply an antiviral activity, if human tumors were indeed caused by virus infections, as seems to be the case with many tumors in animals. The growth of many RNA and DNA tumor viruses is inhibited by interferon treatment; furthermore, cell transformation and tumor induction by agents as diverse as polyoma virus, Rous sarcoma virus, murine sarcoma and leukemia viruses, and *Herpes saimari* virus are also suppressed by interferon treatment. There is, however, no strong evidence that tumors in humans are often, or

TABLE XV. Possible Basis for Antitumor Activity of Interferons

1. Direct inhibition of virus growth
2. Inhibition of tumor cell growth
3. Activation of natural killer cells
4. Macrophage stimulation
5. Increase in histocompatability antigen expression

even rarely caused by virus infections, so that at present there is no reason to think the antitumor action of interferons in humans is an extension of its antiviral activity.

There is, however, one interesting case where interferon is probably effective on humor tumor that is virus induced. In some infants there are recurrent, difficult to treat laryngeal papillomas. These tumors are due to infection by human papillomatoses virus, a human papovavirus that also causes warts. The childhood laryngeal polyps induced by this agent respond very well to interferon treatment according to Strander's group in Sweden and others. It is important to remember that this is probably an antiviral activity; in any case, laryngeal papillomas are not malignant tumors.

The inhibition of chemically or radiation-induced tumors and transplantable tumors does, however suggest that the antitumor action of interferons is due to something more than its antiviral activity. The induction of both methylcholanthrene (a cancer-inducing hydrocarbon) and radiation-induced fibrosarcomas in mice is inhibited by treatment with interferon or interferon inducers. In addition, the growth of transplantable tumors in mice, rabbits, or rats is inhibited by interferons or by interferon inducers.

The transplantation of tumors into immune-deficient nude mice is an especially interesting system in which to study the effects of interferons on tumors. Nude mice accept from other species tumor grafts that then grow rapidly. Since interferons are usually species specific in their antiviral action, it was of great interest to test whether such tumors in nude mice responded to mouse interferon or to interferon of the species from which the tumor was derived. When mice carrying human breast tumors were treated with human or mouse interferon, tumor growth was inhibited only by the human interferon. These results are of some significance, since they strongly suggest that the antitumor action of interferon in these animals must be directed against the tumor itself. It is most unlikely that the mouse immune system responded to human interferon; it is possible, but very unlikely, that the growth of a latent virus in the human breast tumor tissue was inhibited by human interferon treatment. In this system it would appear that the cell growth inhibitory property of interferon is the most important in suppressing tumor growth. The other factors mentioned in Table XV might be more relevant in other systems.

Interferons have also been reported to inhibit cell differentiation in some systems. For instance, high concentrations of mouse interferon (more than 1000 units/ml) inhibited the maturation of Friend leukemia virus-infected cells after dimethylsulfoxide treatment. In these cells growth was slowed and globin synthesis reduced. Interferon treatment also inhibited the conversion of mouse fibroblasts into adipocytes after treatment with insulin; in interferon-treated cells lipid accumulation was markedly slowed. It is very likely that other effects of interferon on cell differentiation will be uncovered.

EFFECTS ON INTRACELLULAR ENZYMES AND OTHER CELL–PRODUCED SUBSTANCES

In addition to the enzyme precursors for protein kinase and $2',5'$-oligoadenylate synthetase expressed during the establishment of antiviral activity, interferons have been reported to cause enhanced production or activity of other enzymes in tissue culture cells (Table XVI). Thus, the induction of arylhydrocarbon hydroxylase by benzanthracene was stimulated by mouse interferon treatment of fetal mouse cells, and interferon treatment of mouse cells resulted in a significant increase in the total level of tRNA methylase activity.

Examples of inhibition by interferons, rather than stimulation, have also been reported, for although the effect of interfer-

TABLE XVI. Interferon Effects on Intracellular Enzymes and Other Cellular Production

Products and enzymes the synthesis of which is increased by interferon treatment:
  Histamine
  Hyaluronic acid
  Prostaglandin E
  tRNA methylase
  Aryl hydrocarbon hydroylase
  Protein kinase
  2′,5′-oligoadenylate synthetase

Enzyme activities inhibited by interferon treatment:
  Tyrosine amino transferase
  Glycerol-3-phosphate dehydrogenase
  Glutamine synthetase
  Ornithine decarboxylase
  S-adenosyl-1-methionine decarboxylase
  UDP-N-acetylglucosamine-dolichol monophosphate transferase

ons in whole cells is less dramatic than that caused by inhibitors of total protein synthesis, several instances have been described indicating the selective inhibition of specific intracellular enzymes by interferons. Pretreatment of cells with mouse or rat interferon resulted in a significant suppression of the dexamethasone-induced tyrosine amino transferase in rat heptoma cells. Similarly, hydrocortisone-induced synthesis of glycerol-3-phosphate dehydrogenase in rat glial cells or glutamine synthetase in chick embryonic retinal cells were inhibited when cells were pretreated with rat or chick interferon, respectively. In addition, the induction of ornithine decarboxylase (ODC), a key enzyme in polyamine biosynthesis in mouse Swiss 3T3 cells was inhibited by mouse interferon treatment. S-Adenosyl-1-methionine decarboxylase (SAM-decarboxylase), another inducible enzyme in the polyamine biosynthesis pathway, can also be inhibited by interferon treatment in 3T3 cells. Interferon treatment inhibits the activity of UDP-N-acetylglucosamine-dolichyl monphosphate transferase in interferon-treated mouse cells, a finding that may be important in several of the activities of interferons, as this enzyme involves the first step in the glycosylation of most glycoproteins. For instance, the inhibitory effect of interferons on the production of viral glycoproteins and some of the actions on the immune system and cell replication might well be related to an inhibition of this enzyme.

In general, there appears to be some selectivity in the types of enzymes inhibited by interferon treatment, since in chick retinal cells the induction of glutamine synthetase was inhibited while the level of enzymes like acetylcholine esterase or lactic dehydrogenase was unaffected. Similarly, although serum induced the synthesis of ODC and glucose transport proteins in quiescent Swiss 3T3 cells, only the former was inhibited by treatment with interferon. The selective inhibition exerted by interferons is further exemplified by the observation that in Friend virus leukemia cells the dimethyl sulfoxide-induced synthesis of globin was inhibited in the absence of any effect on gross protein synthesis, whereas in the case of glycoprotein synthesis-related enzymes, only the transferase for N-acetylglucosamine was inhibited, and the transferases for mannose or glucose were almost unaffected by interferon treatment.

CELL SURFACE ALTERATION

Interferon treatment induces a number of changes in the surface of cells (Table XVII). These changes are of a chemical, physical, morphological, and immunological nature; however, it is not yet established what, if any, relationship they have to the known biological activities of interferons, such as the induction of an antiviral state, modulation of the immune system, or inhibition of cell growth. There are certainly examples of polypeptide hormones and other biologically active molecules that induce intracellular changes by first binding to the cell surfaces and then activating changes on the plasma membrane; these changes in turn result in profound alterations in cell function. What is unknown right now, as far as interferons are concerned, is how changes in the cell surface might result in the types of alterations in Table

TABLE XVII. Changes in the Cell Surface Induced by Interferon Treatment

Alteration in plasma membrane density
Increase in intramembranous particles
Alteration in cell surface charge
Altered capacity to bind thyroid-stimulating hormone or cholera toxin
Increase in binding of concanavalin A
Increase in cytotoxicity of lymphocytes for target cells and in expression of cell
    surface antigens
Altered exposure of surface gangliosides
Increase in intracellular levels of cyclic AMP

XVII. It is also unclear how the alterations of the cell surface themselves are accomplished.

When plasma membrane preparations from mouse cells were analyzed on discontinuous sucrose gradients, in control cells 77% of the plasma membrane banded in sucrose at a density of 1.22–1.23 and 23% at 1.23; in interferon-treated cells, 40% banded at 1.22–1.23 and 60% at 1.23. This probably indicated that the protein-to-lipid ratio was increased in the membranes of interferon-treated cells. Since the main components of intramembranous particles are glycoproteins, these results correlate with those on intramembraneous particles discussed in the next paragraph.

Interferon treatment resulted in an increase in the concentration of intramembraneous particles of mouse cells, a change detected morphologically by freeze-fracture electron microscopy. The number of intramembraneous particles on the fracture faces of the plasma membrane increased from two- to sixfold after interferon treatment for 48 hr. The kinetics of the particle increase followed that of the establishment of antiviral activity, and both intramembraneous particle density and antiviral activity decreased to control levels by 48 hr after the removal of interferon.

Other methods of analysis have suggested that interferon treatment alters the cell surface. When placed in an electric field, interferon-treated mouse cells have a higher electrophoretic mobility toward the anode than did control cells. This result indicated that interferon treatment increases the negative net charge on the cell surface and is consistent with other observations that interferon treatment alters the electrochemical gradient across cell membranes by increasing the net intramembraneous negative charge.

Plasma membranes of interferon-treated mouse cells had an altered capacity to bind thyroid-stimulating hormone (TSH) or cholera toxin. This was consistent with the observation that these substances can inhibit interferon action. ^{125}I-labeled TSH and ^{125}I-labeled cholera toxin can be specifically bound to preparations of mouse L cell plasma membranes, since such binding was prevented by unlabeled thyrotropin or cholera toxin, but not by other polypeptides such as insulin, glucagon, prolactin, growth horomone, human chorionic gonadotropin, or luteinizing hormone. Mouse interferon also inhibited ^{125}I-labeled TSH binding to mouse or human cell plasma membranes. The effect of mouse interferon on ^{125}I-labeled cholera toxin binding was more complex, with inhibition occurring only after an initial enhancement at low interferon concentrations. A concentration of interferon ten times as high was required to inhibit ^{125}I-labeled cholera toxin binding as compared with ^{125}I-labeled TSH binding. Mouse interferon was able to displace bound ^{125}I-labeled TSH. In addition, interferon treatment has been reported to increase the binding of concanavalin A to the surface of murine leukemia L_{1210} cells.

Some of the previously mentioned immunological studies have suggested an alteration in cell surfaces following interferon treatment. This includes the interferon-induced enhancement of the specific cytotoxicity of sensitized mouse lymphocytes. When suspensions of splenic lymphocytes from C57BL/6 mice that had been immunized with L_{1210} cells were incubated with mouse brain interferon or with medium that did not contain interferon, the cells incubated with interferon had enhanced cytotoxic effects against L_{1210} cells. Interferon had no effect on the cytotoxic properties of nonsensitized lymphocytes. The factor responsible for the enhanced cytotoxicity of lymphocytes could not be separated from the antiviral factor in interferon preparations. These results suggested that interferon in this system induced a surface alteration in the splenic lymphocytes, and this alteration increased their cytotoxic properties. Also, as noted earlier, mouse interferon has been shown to enhance the expression of cell surface histocompatibility antigens in L_{1210} cells.

Interferon treatment has also been shown to alter the surface exposure of some gangliosides (glycolipids) and other components of the plasma membrane. The predominant gangliosides in the plasma membranes of interferon-sensitive mouse cells have been implicated as interferon-specific receptor components. No difference in ganglioside pattern could be detected in membranes isolated from mouse cells before or after interferon treatment; however, differences in surface exposure of gangliosides were detected after enzymatic treatment of membranes. This suggested a change in orientation of these gangliosides in the membrane.

Possibly connected with the multiple membrane effects of interferon treatment is the stimulation of cyclic AMP (cAMP) by interferon treatment; however, no definitive effects of interferon on adenylate cyclase, the enzyme that produces cAMP from ATP, have as yet been reported. Thus, the stimulatory effect on cAMP production could arise from nonspecific changes in the plasma membrane. Alternatively, the possibility exists that interferon may be regulating cyclase and cAMP production in a receptor-dependent fashion, as has been reported for several receptors. Functional analogies between interferon and other known receptor-related regulatory patterns would in turn imply a cell surface receptor mechanism for interferon actions. As the functionally related binding of interferon to the cell surface has not yet been elucidated, it would be especially important to carry out studies on possible cyclase alterations in interferon-treated cells.

The findings discussed in this chapter suggest that interferons have a wide spectrum of biological activity. The fact that they were discovered as antiviral substances has in a sense prejudiced how they were considered for a long period of time. Had they been discovered by a cell biologist or an immunologist, it is very likely that their antiviral properties would have remained unknown for many years. At present their role as modifiers of the immune response or as cell growth factors is undergoing intense investigation. It is certainly possible that interferons were originally one of these, but have acquired during evolutionary development the characteristics of extremely active antiviral substances.

BIBLIOGRAPHY

De Maeyer, E., and DeMaeyer, J. (1977). Effect of interferons on cell-mediated immunity. *Tex. Rep. Biol. Med.* **35**, 370–374.

Friedman, R. M. (1979). Interferons: interactions with cell surfaces. *Interferon* **1**, 53–74.

Gresser, I., DeMaeyer-Guignard, J., *et al.* (1979). Electrophoretically pure mouse interferon exerts multiple biologic effects. *Proc. Nat. Acad. Sci. USA* **76**, 5308–5312.

Grollman, E. J., Lee, G., *et al.* (1978). Relationship of the structure and function of the interferon receptor to hormone receptors and establishment of the antiviral state. *Cancer Res.* **38**, 4172–4185.

Johnson, H. M. (1977). Effect of interferon on antibody formation. *Tex. Rep. Biol. Med.* **35**, 357–369.

7

INTERFERONS AND RECOVERY FROM VIRAL INFECTIONS

When interferons were first discovered it seemed likely to Isaacs that such natural antiviral substances might well play a role in recovery from virus infections. This seemed possible for two main reasons, one of which is suggested in Fig. 13, based on a clinical study of volunteers infected with influenza virus. Of the reactions to virus infections studied, interferon production was the earliest. Production of significant amounts of antibodies comes later, possibly too late to alter the outcome of a primary virus infection. No one, of course, argues against the importance of antibodies in preventing secondary virus infections (or reinfections); one has only to note the usefulness of innoculation with vaccines for preventing smallpox, poliomyelitis, measles, mumps, and rubella virus infections. All of these vaccines induce antiviral antibodies. The slowness of the antibody response, however, seemed to indicate that some natural factor other than antibodies could be called into play very early in primary virus infections and that factor might well be interferon.

One other finding that suggested additional responses were involved in recovery from primary virus infections was the discovery of agammaglobulinemia. In this congenital or acquired disease, the patients, who are unable to produce significant titers of antibodies, are subject to recurrent severe bacterial infections; in fact, the discovery of this condition had to await the era of antibiotics, because before then the death of agammaglobulinemics was probably lost in the general background of infant deaths

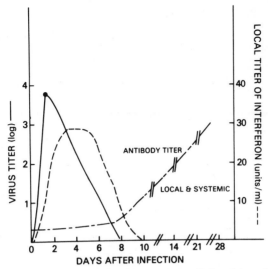

Fig. 13. Infection of humans with influenza virus: Role of interferons or anti-body in the recovery process.

In human volunteers infected with influenza or other upper respiratory viruses virus titers in the nasal tissue rapidly rise (solid line). They reach a peak by 2–3 days after infection and then rapidly decline. Local and systemic antibody titers (–––––––) start to rise about 5–7 days after infection. Interferon titers (–––) rise rapidly with the virus infection and fall with elimination of virus from the upper respiratory tract. (Based on data from human volunteer studies on infection of the upper respiratory tract by viruses.)

caused by infectious diseases. At any rate, a remarkable observation was that agammaglobulinemic patients usually recovered from primary virus infections about as well as did normal people. This had to mean that antibody production alone did not explain recovery from primary virus diseases.

In order to understand how interferons can help in the recovery from virus infections, it would be important to review briefly the development of these diseases. In general, there are two types of virus diseases, the first of which is illustrated by the course of influenza virus infection (Fig. 13). Disease caused by influenza viruses is generally localized to the site of primary infection, the upper respiratory tract. This is true of most other viruses that cause upper respiratory infections such as colds or of gastrointestinal diseases caused by viruses. Influenza viruses can, of course, cause severe pneumonia, but this is unusual in humans.

Therefore, the disease associated with influenza virus infection is caused by local multiplication of the virus and is a compound effect caused by the cell damage by the virus and by the response of the host. Any meaningful response to such an infection must be very rapid. As indicated in Fig. 13, the production of antibody is generally too slow to account for the fall in virus titers in the tissues of the upper respiratory tract, whereas the rise in interferon titer does seem to correlate better. It is, therefore, not unlikely that interferons could play a role in the recovery from primary infections where the disease is associated with virus replication at the site of infection.

In most diseases caused by viruses, however, the primary site of infection is not the locus of the disease usually associated with that particular virus infection. To use an unfamiliar example, Fig. 14 traces the course of a typical mosquito-borne encephalitis. Virus is picked up by the insect biting an infected animal or human and multiplies in the gut of the mosquito; infection is passed on by a bite to a new victim. The virus multiplies in the local tissues and spreads to local lymph nodes and then to organs

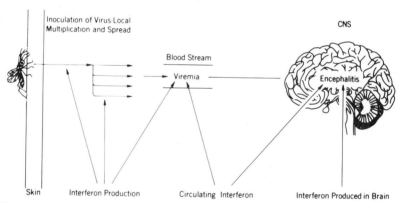

Fig. 14. Course of an arbovirus infection in an animal. Role of interferon in the recovery process.

The skin of a human is being bitten by a mosquito. The virus is deposited at this site but spreads locally; local interferon production is induced. The virus that survives multiplies extensively and enters the bloodstream, causing a viremia, fever, and chills. The viremia in turn induces an interferonemia (circulating interferon). If the virus titer is not reduced sufficiently, residual virus may enter the central nervous system (CNS), the target organ for these viruses, and cause an encephalitis. Even here, interferon production takes place; this may act to control virus spread in the brain.

such as the liver and the spleen; it is finally released into the blood to cause a viremia that serves two purposes from the point of view of the virus: the first is to permit mosquitos a chance to pick up and propagate the virus; the second is to enter the virus target organ, the central nervous system, where virus replication can go on relatively unimpeded by the immune system and, incidentally (as far as the virus is concerned), where it can result in severe illness or death of the patient.

Interferon is induced at several points in this replication cycle. Interferons are produced at the local site of infection, and as the virus spreads, they are released into the blood to cause an interferonemia that often coincides with the viremia caused by the infection (Fig. 9). Both local interferon production and interferonemia may by decreasing virus production contribute to protection against infection in the target organ, in this case the brain.

The mosquito-borne encephalitis used as an illustration is by no means atypical of virus diseases. Other examples that seem to follow the same pattern are listed in Table XVIII. In such diseases interferon production may well contribute to a limitation of the virus infection.

Between death and complete recovery from a virus infection there is one alternative condition, a state of chronic infection. There are several diseases that are suspected of being related to such infections. The first category includes chronic hepatitis B infection and progressive multifocal leukoencephalopathy. Other

TABLE XVIII. Site of Primary Infection and Target Organs of Various Virus Infections

Virus	Primary infection	Typical target organ
Hepatitis A	Gastrointestinal tract	Liver
Poliomyelitis	Gastrointestinal tract	Central nervous system
Measles	Respiratory tract	Skin
Mumps	Respiratory tract	Salivary glands
Hepatitis B	Subcutaneous tissues (needle stick)	Liver
Rabies	Subcutaneous tissues (animal bite)	Central nervous system
Smallpox	Respiratory tract	Skin and other organs

diseases that certainly appear to be due to chronic virus infections are subacute sclerosing panencephalitis, Creutzfeldt-Jakob disease, Kuru, and perhaps, multiple sclerosis.

Because the experimental animal models involved in these chronic diseases often involve viruses that are extremely slow growing, much of our understanding of these systems comes from studies carried out in tissue culture systems. At least three factors seem to be involved in establishing and maintaining such chronic infections in tissue cultures. In some cases defective interfering virus particles are produced; this mechanism has been identified as active in a chronic infection with vesicular stomatitis virus. In such an infection particles with truncated viral RNA are produced; these defective virus particles absorb to cells, whereupon the shortened viral RNA enters the cell and proceeds to interfere with the replication of full-length viral RNA—thus the name *defective interfering particles.*

In other chronic infections, especially those with paramyxoviruses and rhabdoviruses, temperature-sensitive mutants of the infecting agent are rapidly produced and act as interfering agents for wild-type virus replication. This appears to be an important mechanism for the propagation of chronically infected cultures, although it is unclear how the temperature-sensitive mutants are generated or why they should be so efficient at interfering with the wild-type parental strain.

The production of interferon seems to be a third important mechanism in establishing and maintaining chronic viral infections in tissue culture, although so far it has usually been reported to be active only in conjunction with the generation of temperature-sensitive mutants. How these interact is so far unknown, although likely mechanisms of action may be the generation of higher titers of interferon by temperature-sensitive mutants than by wild-type viruses, and the rapid evolution of temperature-sensitive mutants in the presence of low titers of interferon.

Whether these three mechanisms are relevant to chronic virus infections in man and animals is at present unknown, but it is possible that interferon production will figure as a factor in the chronic infections mentioned earlier. Certainly, studies in tissue culture will be helpful in elucidating how such infections may be established and maintained.

EVIDENCE THAT INTERFERONS ARE ACTIVE FACTORS IN THE RECOVERY FROM PRIMARY VIRUS INFECTIONS

Table XIX summarizes evidence that interferons can contribute to recovery from primary virus infections. In many infections that have been studied in animals and man, production of interferons very early in infection has been demonstrated (see Fig. 13 for one example). This means that interferons appear early in the infectious cycle and have an opportunity to start inducing antiviral activity before the infection has had a chance to spread. This is indeed a prerequisite for a substance to be effective—it must be present early. It is, however, only part of the requirement for effectiveness: not only must interferons be present early, but they must be present in sufficient quantities to account for recovery from infections.

There are indeed many studies of interferon production in which sufficient titers are produced to suggest that there is enough activity to contribute to the recovery process. Most of these studies are based on blood interferon levels or on titers of interferon in an organ. Even though such results are impressive enough, it is interesting to consider how high levels of interferon must be at the

TABLE XIX. Evidence That Interferons Contribute to Recovery from Primary Virus Infections

1. Interferons are produced at the site of virus infections quite early in the infection
2. Interferons are produced in sufficient quantity to account for recovery from primary infections
3. Inhibition of interferon production increases the severity of viral infections
4. Administration of exogenous interferon inhibits the development of viral infections

immediate site of a virus infection. Estimates based on interferon production in tissue culture or in animals suggest that local titers of several thousand units per ml are not only possible but quite likely. Even though interferons must rapidly diffuse from their production site, the high titers achieved locally, even temporarily, may be meaningful, because initiation of antiviral activity takes very little time. It is therefore possible that the high titers of interferon reached temporarily in tissues persist long enough to establish high enough levels of intracellular antiviral activity to contribute significantly to the recovery process. Therefore, tissue-bound beta interferon may be useful in some clinical situations.

Additional evidence that reinforces the theory that interferons are important in recovery from primary virus infections is that in the absence of interferon, viral infections become more severe. As far as is known, there is no natural state in animals where interferon is not produced or where an animal is unresponsive to its own interferon; indeed, in the absence of effective forms of antiviral chemotherapy, such conditions might be incompatible with prolonged survival. One state that does to an extent mimic such a condition is found in the early chick embryo, which is unable to produce interferon until after it is about 1 week old. Such early chick embryos are susceptible to many viruses that grow to higher titers than they do in older embryos.

A somewhat more convincing system, as far as establishing the importance of interferons in recovery from virus infections, has been used by Gresser and his associates, who have obtained the services of a sheep that has the capacity to produce large quantities of antibody to mouse interferon. They have treated mice with this antiserum before and during infection with several viruses. Results of these studies clearly indicated that in most cases viral infections were increased in severity in these animals. Death was more rapid and the 50% lethal dose of virus was significantly decreased in the mice treated with antibody to mouse interferon. Such experiments strongly suggest that interferon is important in the normal recovery process.

Another experiment that can be performed is to test whether exogenous interferon significantly aids in the recovery of animals from acute virus infections. Such studies have been carried out in monkeys, chicks, hamsters, guinea pigs, rats, mice, and rabbits infected with examples of most of the group of RNA or DNA viruses commonly employed in studying infections in the laboratory. The results of such studies have often shown impressive increases in survival and increased 50% lethal doses of virus in animals treated with interferons.

This evidence strongly suggests an important role for interferon in recovery from primary virus infections. Further evidence that this conclusion is valid is that viruses causing attenuated infections are sometimes better inducers of, or more sensitive to interferons than are viruses causing serious infections. This has proved to be so with strains from several diverse groups of viruses such as Newcastle disease, Semliki Forest, foot and mouth disease, and rubella viruses, although there are certainly strains of viruses in which attenuation appears unrelated to interferon production or action. In addition, effective rabies vaccines in post exposure treatment (that is, after an animal bite) are those that induce interferon production; those that are not effective do not induce interferon. Interferon, therefore, assists in developing protection against rabies.

INTERACTIONS BETWEEN INTERFERONS AND OTHER NATURAL ANTIVIRAL MECHANISMS

Although the antiviral activity of interferons is indeed important in recovery from some primary viral infections, there are other mechanisms that seem to play roles of varying importance in recovery from different viral diseases. Cell-mediated immunity is thought to act as an antiviral mechanism since viruses that alter the plasma membrane by insertion of viral proteins bring about changes that make these cells targets for natural killer (NK) or killer (K) cell lysis. This mechanism is therefore likely to be important in infections with herpesviruses and viruses that alter the cell surfaces so that they can bud from it. This would include such agents as influenza virus, paramyxoviruses, most arthropod-borne viruses, and RNA tumor viruses.

97

The febrile response also seems to play a role in recovery from some virus infections. Many wild-type viruses do not grow as well at 40°C as they do at body temperature, 37°C; indeed, some attenuated virus strains act as temperature-sensitive mutants. Elevation of body temperature or local increases in temperature, such as is seen in an area of inflammation, may therefore serve as a potent antiviral mechanism.

Other aspects of the inflammatory response may also act as significant antiviral factors. For instance, during the inflammatory reaction, acid products are generated and the pH is often lowered locally. Also, white blood cells and tissue monocytes are brought into the area of infection during the inflammatory reaction. The granulocytes and monocytes provide phagocytic activity that may be quite important in engulfing viruses and thus removing them from the site of infection, if the phagocytic cell is capable of killing the virus.

The inflammatory response and the febrile reaction may also act to hasten the antibody response and to increase the level of antibody produced. This may prove of importance in infections in which antibody is thought to play a role in recovery.

It is interesting to note that all of the mechanisms discussed, such as fever, phagocytosis, inflammation, and cell-mediated immunity, were originally considered to be quite independent of one another and of the interferon mechanism in acting to aid recovery from virus infection. As some of the nonantiviral activities of interferons have come to light, it has become apparent that interferons may stimulate many mechanisms that were previously thought to be independent (Table XX).

For instance, interferons stimulate the phagocytic activity of macrophages, an activity that may result in the destruction of infecting viruses. Antibody production itself can under some conditions be stimulated by interferon treatment, when low concentrations of interferon are employed or when interferon appears after viral antigen, certainly the sequence that occurs during infections with viruses. In addition, some investigators have reported that interferons directly or indirectly stimulate the inflammatory and the febrile responses. Finally, some aspects of the cell-mediated immune response, which are stimulated by interferon, may play

TABLE XX. Interaction of Various Antiviral Mechanisms with Interferons

Mechanism	Action of interferon
Phagocytosis by macrophages	Stimulated
Antibody production	Stimulated by low concentration and late administration
Inflammatory response	Stimulated
Fever	Induced
Cell-mediated immunity; NK and K cell-mediated lysis of infected cells	Stimulated

an important role in recovery from viral infections. This includes the stimulation of cell lysis by killer and natural killer cells, activities that can be directed against infected cells in which the plasma membrane has been altered by viral infection. It is possible that the action of interferon to prevent murine RNA tumor viruses from budding off the cell surface has the same effect, in that a cell surface that has so much viral antigen associated with it is likely to interest surveillance cells with which the immune system monitors for the presence in the body of foreign antigens.

Without attempting to overplay the importance that interferons may have in recovery from primary virus infections, the interactions with the other systems discussed earlier provide additional, convincing evidence of a significant role for interferons. Therefore, Isaacs' original notions about interferons and the pathogenesis of viral diseases were probably right on the mark.

"INTERFERONS ARE A GOOD THING, BUT TOO MUCH OF A GOOD THING CAN BE A BAD THING"

The title of this section is a quote from a talk given by Dr. Ion Gresser on the role of interferons in the pathogenesis of disease due to infection with the arenavirus lymphocytic choriomeningitis virus (LCMV). These findings may have some implications for human diseases caused by members of this virus group.

99

LCMV has long been known to cause two sorts of diseases in mice. The first is a rapidly fatal form of meningitis in adult mice; the second is related to the establishment of a chronic state of infection in which high titers of virus are present in the mouse blood and tissues. The mice with chronic infections are inoculated at birth with virus; after about 6 months, such mice develop a chronic renal disease, glomerulonephritis. Immune complexes consisting of complement, LCMV, and antibody to LCMV have been reported in the glomerular basement membrane of these mice; therefore, it was assumed that such complexes were related to the pathogenesis of the renal disease associated with chronic LCMV infection.

Some doubt was shed on the significance of these findings by studies involving the administration of antibody to mouse interferon at the time of infection of newborn mice with LCMV. The mice that had received the antibody to interferon did better than did controls, in spite of the fact that there were high titers of LCMV in the mice receiving the anti-interferon antibody. One possible interpretation of this result was that interferon production induced by LCMV infection had something to do with the pathogenesis of the late renal disease. To determine whether this was a reasonable possibility, newborn mice infected with LCMV were checked for interferon production; indeed, these mice were found to have high titers of circulating interferon. The next step was to inject newborn mice with interferon in order to check whether interferon itself could cause the renal disease. The mice receiving interferon did develop glomerulonephitis at about the same time as did the mice injected with LCMV at birth. This study therefore suggests that late renal disease may result from production of high titers of interferon in newborn mice. Subsequent work has indicated that the pathogenesis of attenuated LCMV strains is related to their ability to induce the production of interferon; those strains of virus that are better interferon inducers are more virulent. It has also been noted that treatment with an interferon inducer of monkeys infected with arenaviruses results in exacerbation of disease rather than its mitigation.

It is therefore possible that with some viruses too much interferon at the wrong time might indeed be a bad thing.

BIBLIOGRAPHY

Baron, S. (1973). The defensive and biological roles of the interferon system. *In* "Interferons and Interferon Inducers" (Finter, N. B., ed.). Amer. Elsevier, New York. pp. 267–293.

Friedman, R. M., and Ramseur, J. M. (1979). Mechanisms of persistent infections by cytopathic viruses in tissue culture. Brief review. *Arch. Virol.* **60**, 83–103.

Reviere, Y., Gresser, I., *et al.* (1977). Inhibition by anti-interferon serum of lymphocytic choriomeningitis virus disease in suckling mice. *Proc. Nat. Acad. Sci. USA* **74**, 2135–2139.

Yabrov, A. A. (1980). Interferon and non-specific resistance. Human Sci. Press, New York.

8

CLINICAL USES
OF INTERFERONS

There are several human disease conditions in which interferon therapy may prove to be useful. The treatment of viral infections (Tables XXI and XXII) is an obvious application because of the efficiency of interferons as natural antiviral substances. In addition, interferons may prove useful in the therapy of human cancers. This statement is based on the cell growth inhibitory properties of interferons, their effects on the immune system, and on the extensive work that points to direct inhibitory action of interferons on tumor growth in mice and other animals. Finally, although no studies with this in mind have so far been carried out, the immunoregulatory effects of interferons suggest they may be of use in some human disease conditions caused by malfunction of the immune response.

PHARMACOLOGY OF INTERFERONS IN HUMANS

Interferons are usually administered to patients at dose levels of $3-10 \times 10^6$ units per day. At present P–IF (partially purified interferon of leukocyte origin, see later discussion) interferon preparations of Cantell contains 10^5-10^6 international interferon units per milligram of protein and thus are far less than 1% interferon. There is general agreement that only interferon preparations with at least 10^6 units per milligram protein should be used.

TABLE XXI. Viral Infections with Potential for Interferon Therapy

1. Chronic hepatitis B infection
2. Herpesvirus infections (ocular, local, or systemic)
3. Influenza and other respiratory tract virus infections
4. Rabies and other viral zoonoses
5. Arbovirus infections (e.g., Eastern equine encephalitis)
6. Slow virus diseases (Kuru, subacute sclerosing panencephalitis, Creutzfelt–Jakob disease, etc.)

When a preparation such as this is administered intravenously, the interferon is rapidly cleared from the blood; therefore, intramuscular administration is the usual form of interferon therapy. Intramuscular inoculation of 3–10 × 10⁶ units of P–IF results in circulating human interferon titers of 100–1,000 units for about 24 hr. This means that significant amounts of interferon are present in most body fluids until the next dose is administered. In considering these figures it should be noted, however, that interferon action is not immediately reversed by a drop in the titer of interferon, since antiviral activity persists for many hours after interferon is removed; therefore, the maintenance of high interferon titers may not be as important as it seems. Intramuscular injection of beta human interferon may not be helpful because of the propensity of this interferon to stick to tissues, thus failing to enter the circulation readily, although this property might be useful for local treatment because interferon will stay at the injection site. So far, there have been no studies in man with gamma interferon, but because of some of its unique properties, gamma interferon may prove to be very useful clinically.

As suggested earlier, serum levels of interferon do not pro-

TABLE XXII. Viral Infections with Potential for Therapy with Interferons in Immunocompromised Patients

1. *Herpes zoster* and *varicella* (VZ)
2. Cytomegalovirus
3. Epstein-Barr virus (EBV) infections
4. *Herpes simplex* infections
5. Rubella (congenital)
6. Progressive multifocal leukoencephalopathy

vide information about interferon levels in all the extracellular fluids; indeed, it is even possible that the titer of interferon is interstitial fluids significantly differs from serum levels. The level in cerebrospinal fluid, and thus the brain, is, however, definitely lower than in the blood when interferons are administered intramuscularly or intravenously, since interferons do not cross the blood–brain barrier. It is possible that this barrier may not be significant in the course of an inflammatory disease of the brain such as a viral meningitis or encephalitis. In such conditions, the levels of interferons in the brain may come close to that in the blood. At any rate, it is certainly feasible to administer interferons directly into the cerebrospinal fluid to get high local titers; this might indeed by a useful way to attempt to treat viral diseases or malignant tumors of the central nervous system.

In addition, interferons do not appear to pass through the placental barrier. This might be of importance in conditions like rubella infection, where a maternal virus infection attacks the embryo, causing subsequent severe congenital anomalies in the resulting newborn. Neither the maternal interferon response nor administration of interferon or interferon inducers to the mother would be expected to help the fetus much just because interferons do not enter the fetal circulation.

Circulating interferons appear to be eliminated in the kidney and the liver. In the kidney, interferons are filtered in the glomeruli but are for the most part resorbed in the tubular apparatus. In the liver, interferon catabolism appears to depend on removal of terminal sialic acid residues in the interferon molecule so that the carbohydrates galactose and fructose are exposed. In the perfused liver, therefore, interferon is first catabolized at a slow rate; then the process accelerates. If almost all carbohydrate is removed from an interferon, its catabolism is not accelerated. This is especially important in considering the possible clinical usefulness of human interferons derived from human genes cloned in microorganisms. Interferons thus produced an unglycosylated, so that it is comforting to know that they will probably be biologically active *in vivo*.

Discussion of the pharmacology of interferons and their glycosylation leads to several important questions. Among these are: What is the role of the carbohydrate on some interferons? Can the interferon molecule be modified in some manner so that its catabolism is slowed up in the body? The answer to the first question is not known, although, like many glycoproteins, it would seem that the carbohydrate is not required for biological activity. The glycosylation of interferons may, therefore, be necessary to protect the interferon in an intracellular location or after the production of an interferon, to ensure that it gets to its proper location in the cell. As to the second question, it may well be possible to modify interferons to slow up their turnover rate in the body. This has been accomplished for several drugs; it is a modification that may be especially feasible in interferon produced by microorganisms.

Since interferons are natural products, it was originally thought that they would be nontoxic in therapeutic concentration; therefore, the toxic effects seen in patients treated with interferons were at first considered to be due to the impurities present in the preparations employed. However, many natural biological products can be quite toxic in therapeutic doses; consider the adrenal steroids as an example. The so-called side effects of the steroids can be very significant. It is now considered likely that many of the side effects of interferon treatment are due to the interferon itself, a not unreasonable conclusion, because of the very active biological nature of interferons. The important toxic effects so far noted are leukopenia, thrombocytopenia, hair loss, fever, pain, and fatigue, all of which are reversible upon cessation of interferon treatment. The first three listed effects could well be due to the inhibitory effect of interferons on cell growth. It is likely that additional toxic effects will be noted as use of interferons in humans increases.

INTERFERON PREPARATIONS AVAILABLE FOR USE IN HUMANS

At the time of this writing, there are very few preparations of interferon available for use in humans. Most clinical studies with human interferons have employed preparations from leukocytes that contain alpha (99%) and beta (about 1%) interferons. As noted in Chapter 4, these have been made in the laboratory of Kari Cantell at the Finnish Red Cross in Helsinki by stimulation with Sendai virus of the pooled buffy coat white cells from donated blood. The interferon obtained is partially purified by precipitation with KSCN and ethanol, yielding preparations (P-IF) with specific activities of at most 10^6 units of interferon per milligram of protein. Each buffy coat yields about 10^6 units of interferon. The cost is $20–50 per 10^6 units at present.

In addition, some clinical studies have employed preparations of diploid human fibroblast interferon. This is produced from well-characterized lines of human foreskin cells, for example, by stimulating monolayers with polyIC and using superinduction techniques, such as the addition of cycloheximide and actinomycin D. These preparations contain only beta-type interferon. The specific activities of the fibroblast interferons obtained so far are low, about 6×10^4 units per milligram of protein, but rapid progress in the purification of such preparations is being made.

The other source of interferon at present is preparations from Namalva lymphoblastoid cells. These cells can be stimulated to produce high titers of alpha (about 80%) and beta (20%) interferons by paramyxoviruses; however, lymphoblastoid cells contain part or all of the Epstein–Barr virus (EBV) genome and Namalva cells are derived from a lymphoma. The interferon produced by them requires, therefore, extensive investigation and purification but may prove to be less expensive than are interferons from leukocyte or fibroblast sources.

Of the interferons available, as noted earlier, most of our clinical experience has been gained employing interferon prepared from leukocytes. We therefore know that at least this form of interferon is effective in some clinical diseases (see later discussion). Although the tendency for beta interferons to stick to tissues may limit their usefulness, intravenous injection of beta interferon may prove to be a feasible method of therapy if such preparations can be purified to a sufficient degree. If Namalva interferon were sufficiently purified, it too might be generally useful in humans, for as previously noted, to limit the use of purified lymphoblastoid interferon only to the treatment of tumors may be overcautious.

The two important problems associated with all the interferon preparations in use are their limited supply and their high cost of production. Both problems will require great expertise to solve. The use of cloning techniques may go a long way in solving the supply problem. If it should not prove feasible to employ in the clinic human interferon produced in microorganisms, it will still be possible to augment greatly interferon production. Almost all the clinical work on human interferon has employed the production facilities of Dr. Cantell at the Finnish Red Cross, so that all the rest of the huge quantity of blood donated in the world is in effect wasted as far as interferon production goes. As noted earlier, if even a small fraction of this potential could be harnessed, our supply of useful human interferon from leukocytes would be enormously increased. The methods developed by Cantell are quite general and should be adaptable to large blood collection centers willing to spend the time to attempt to use his techniques. It might also be possible to develop simple methods to produce large quantities of purified human beta interferon from mass fibroblast or other cultures.

Costs for interferon production will fall as its production rises. Should interferons prove to be clinically useful for relatively common human disease conditions, it follows that it will become cheaper as advantage is taken of mass methods of production. Therefore, solving the problems of usefulness and availability of human interferon will necessarily greatly contribute to the solution of the cost problem.

CLINICAL USES OF HUMAN INTERFERONS

Viral Diseases in the Normal Host (Table XXI)

Several virus infections in humans with normal immune responses might be treated with interferon. In some cases there is experimental evidence that interferon therapy might be of some clinical use (chronic hepatitis B, ocular herpesvirus, and respiratory tract virus infections); in others, the usefulness of interferon is entirely speculative.

Chronic infection with hepatitis B virus can be a serious disease for the affected individual, but it also represents an important public health hazard. The disease is much more frequent and severe in males. In studies at Stanford University in which human leukocyte interferon has been given parenterally to six females with chronic hepatitis B virus infection, two patients completely eliminated all markers for the virus and developed improved liver biopsies. Two other courses of therapy resulted in elimination of Dane particles, the virus, from the circulation, but in a less dramatic improvement in other parameters of chronic hepatitis B virus infection. Three courses of interferon therapy in women resulted in little or no improvement. In males, unfortunately, very little improvement was noted on treatment with interferon alone; however, addition of the antiviral drug adenine arabinoside (Ara-A) to the therapeutic regimen did result in some clinical improvement in 8 of 21 courses of treatment in male patients. In some other clinical centers there has been less success reported in the treatment of this disease with interferon. It is obvious that more controlled clinical studies with combinations of interferon and other antiviral substances are mandatory before any assessment can be made of the role of interferon in the therapy of this disease.

Herpesvirus infections have also been treated with interferons. Experimental *Herpes simplex* keratitis in monkeys responds to local administration of human alpha or beta interferon. In humans, on the other hand, good results were obtained in herpesvirus keratitis only when interferon therapy was combined with thermocautery, debridement, or the antiviral drug trifluorothymidine (TFT); the combination of interferon and TFT appears to be quite promising as a form of therapy. Other studies with *Herpes simplex* infections have shown that reactivation of a chronic herpesvirus labialis following surgical treatment of trigeminal nerve neuralgia can be inhibited by treatment with human leukocyte interferon before surgery. The latter study does suggest that interferons may be useful adjunct in the therapy of herpesvirus infections more severe than reactivation of herpes labialis. More well-controlled clinical studies are in order here too.

Another group of virus diseases in which therapy with interferon may prove useful is respiratory virus infections. In one study leukocyte interferon administered by intranasal spray protected volunteers against colds caused by rhinovirus 4. High doses of interferon had to be administered repeatedly in order to see any positive effect in this study, apparently because of the barrier put up by mucus and the action of the nasal cilia. If these formidable problems can be overcome and topical interferon treatment can be made effective for human respiratory tract infections, there will certainly be a great market for interferon, as the large variety of respiratory viruses that cause disease in man just about precludes the development of a generally effective vaccine for this group of infections.

Rabies is also a disease whose course interferon treatment might favorably affect. After an animal bite, there is often a prolonged incubation period before disease is manifest; indeed, even in symptomatic patients there is a period during which interferon treatment may allow survival of a patient by eliminating the infecting virus, for rabies virus is sensitive to interferon treatment. Curiously, the effectiveness of some rabies vaccines may correlate better with their ability to induce interferon than with their ability to induce antirabies antibodies. It may be that eventually rabies vaccine, intensive care, interferon inducers, and interferon will all play a role in the prevention and treatment of rabies infection. In the case of other zoonoses such as Lassa fever, in which very high mortality is the rule, interferon should be tried as a form of therapy and as a prophylactic treatment for those exposed to the virus. In such cases, interferon treatment might make the difference between life and death, since no therapy is now known for such patients.

Arthropod-borne virus (arbovirus) infections often occur in circumscribed areas in which the disease may be devastating, since these viruses can cause high morbidity and mortality rates. Although there is no evidence that treatment with interferon might prevent or attenuate arbovirus-caused diseases in humans, it would be rational to attempt to treat or prevent arbovirus infections with interferon, because some viruses in this group are among the most interferon-sensitive viruses known, and interferon has proved to be effective in animal studies on arbovirus infections.

Finally, in the absence of any useful form of treatment, it would be reasonable to attempt therapy with interferon in chronic virus infections such as those listed in Table XXI and other diseases such as multiple sclerosis that might have a viral origin. It will probably be extremely difficult to judge whether interferon (or any other) treatment is effective in such disease states because of their slowly progressive nature. In view of the grave outcome of these diseases, however, a trial with interferon could well be justified.

Infectious Diseases in Immunocompromised Patients (Table XX)

Reports on the chronic use of interferon to treat tumor patients suggested that such treatment decreased the incidence and severity of herpes zoster infections in this group. When a study of *varicella–zoster* (VZ) infections in leukemia and lymphoma patients was carried out, it demonstrated that prompt therapy with interferon is an effective form of treatment for VZ infections in this group (Table XXIII). The interferon-treated patients had fewer new lesions, less cutaneous and visceral spread of the disease, decreased pain at primary infection sites, and fewer instances of postherpetic neuralgia than did control patients. The results were significant and suggested that interferon alone or together with other antiviral agents is an effective therapy for this

TABLE XXIII. Results with Interferon Treatment of Early Acute *Herpes zoster* Infection in Lymphoma Patients

Prevention of new local lesions
Prevention of distant cutaneous spread
Less visceral spread
Decreased pain at primary infection site
Decreased frequency and duration of postherpetic neuralgia

virus infection in immunocompromised patients, where its consequences may be grave.

Infections with human cytomegalvirus (CMV), *Herpes simplex* virus (HSV), and the Epstein–Barr virus (EBV) are important in immunosuppressed recipients of kidney and other transplants. Infections with these viruses may be lethal in some cases and in others may contribute to the rejection of the transplant. It was therefore of some significance to determine whether treatment with interferon would reduce the incidence of infection with these viruses. In one study using leukocyte interferon, the treatment reduced the incidence of both CMV and HSV infections and delayed CMV shedding. Such effects might be important in controlling infections in transplantation patients.

In addition, it is possible that the immunosuppressive effects of interferon might help to prevent the early rejection of a transplant, thus providing an additional rationale for its use. It is therefore important that more work be carried out on the effect of interferon treatment on viral infections in transplant patients, both to establish whether this is an effective adjunct to transplantation surgery and to provide information on whether virus infections contribute to rejection of organ transplants.

Interferon treatment has also been shown to effect a transient inhibition of the persistent virus excretion in neonates with congenital rubella virus or CMV infection. It is likely that some other modality of therapy together with interferon may have to be employed to treat congenital infections with CMV or rubella virus, because results with interferon alone have only been suggestive of a positive effect. One interesting observation made on the neonates treated with interferon was their failure to thrive during the treatment, a bit reminiscent of the severe toxic effect of interferon treatment on newborn mice. Obviously, interferon therapy in the neonate will have to be carefully monitored.

One other virus infection that may well be worth attempting to treat in the immunocompromised patient is progressive multifocal leukoencephalophy (PML). This severe neurological disease, which is seen in some treated tumor patients, is caused by a papovavirus related to SV40, a virus whose replication can be inhibited by interferon treatment. Again, because there is little or nothing else to offer patients with PML, it is probably justified to attempt therapy with interferon.

TREATMENT OF HUMAN CANCER
WITH INTERFERON

Table XV lists the reasons why interferon may be an effective treatment for some forms of human cancer. In addition, it should again be emphasized that the work of several laboratories has demonstrated an antitumor effect of interferon treatment in animals; this provides a rationale for attempting such clinical studies in humans. At the time of this writing, however, it is uncertain what, if any, role interferon therapy will play in our armamentarium of anticancer therapy.

A number of human cancers are currently being treated with human interferons, most frequently interferon from human leukocytes. The first study of any size is presently being carried out on osteogenic sarcoma patients at the Karolinska Hospital in Stockholm. Although this is an uncontrolled test of interferon, the results are suggestive of an inhibitory effect of interferon treatment on the spread of the tumor. They have in turn sparked the enthusiasm that has led to the trials of interferon in the other studies listed in Table XXIV.

In the case of nodular poorly differentiated lymphomas, three patients appeared to undergo some clinical improvement and tumor regression while on treatment with interferon; however, this is a capricious disease, one whose progress is notoriously difficult to evaluate. The results of interferon studies on the growth of the other tumors listed in Table XXIV are marginal or negative or, if positive, are positive on so few patients they cannot at present be considered significant. It may well be that interferons will find a place in the therapy of tumors as an adjunct to other forms of treatment, but at present it is difficult to imagine that interferons will be a panacea for human cancer.

One form of tumor deserves repeated comment insofar as interferon treatment is concerned. Laryngeal papillomas respond

TABLE XXIV. Human Tumors in Which Treatment with Interferon Is Being Attempted (as of Fall, 1980)

Osteogenic sarcoma
Multiple myeloma
Hodgkin's disease
Nodular, poorly differentiated lymphoma
Acute lymphocytic leukemia
Chronic lymphocytic leukemia
Breast carcinoma
Melanoma
Nasopharyngeal carcinoma
Laryngeal papilloma[a]

[a] This is a tumor caused by a human papillomatosis virus, but it is *not* a cancer.

very well indeed to systemic treatment with interferon; however, as mentioned in Chapter 6, these tumors are not cancers. They are, like human warts, caused by a human papillomatosis virus. Their response to therapy with interferons is not, therefore, entirely unexpected, nor should it be cited as an example of the successful treatment of a human cancer by interferon.

BIBLIOGRAPHY

Cantell, K. (1979). Why is interferon not in clinical use today? *Interferon* **1**, 1–28.

Cheeseman, S. H., Rubin, R. H., *et al.* (1979). Controlled clinical trial of prophylactic human-leukocyte interferon in renal transplantation. Effects on cytomegalovirus and herpes simplex virus infections. *New Engl. J. Med.* **300**, 1345–1349.

Greenberg, H. B., Pollard, R. B. *et al.* (1976). Human leukocyte interferon and hepatitis B virus infection. *New Engl. J. Med.* **295**, 517–520.

Merigan, T. C., Sikora, K., *et al.* (1978). Preliminary observations on the effect of human leukocyte interferon in non-Hodgkin's lymphoma. *New Engl. J. Med.* **299**, 1449–1453.

Pazin, G. J., Armstrong, J. A., *et al.* (1979). Prevention of reactivated herpes simplex infection by human leukocyte interferon after operation on the trigeminal root. *New Engl. J. Med.* **301**, 225–230.

Strander, H., Adamson, V., *et al.* (1978). Adjuvant interferon treatment of human osteogenic sarcoma. Recent results. *Cancer Res.* **68**, 40–44.

9

THE FUTURE
OF INTERFERONS

It is probably unwise to attempt to write a chapter with this title, as the future in biological sciences can be very unpredictable. It is nevertheless of interest to try to assess where we may be going.

The key to the medical use of interferons is obviously to obtain enough of it to attempt meaningful clinical trials. As of now, of course, such supplies are not available, but there is reason to be sanguine about our prospects in this area. The unexpectedly rapid progress that has been made in the cloning of the human alpha and beta interferon genes gives some cause for this optimism insofar as it makes it seem that the availability of an adequate supply of human interferons in clinical testing is not an impossible dream. As of this writing, none of the interferon produced by this method has been used in trials in humans; however, its antiviral activity in tissue culture systems and in nonhuman primates indicates that it will almost certainly be active in humans. There is the possibility that it may take some time to develop enough human interferon from this source for clinical trials in the near future. If this should be the case, production of interferons by human leukocytes, fibroblasts, or lymphoblastoid cells may be increased to an extent that will permit the necessary studies to be carried out.

In this context, "necessary studies" refers chiefly to the possible use of interferons in the treatment of human cancers. The supplies of human interferons are at present so pitifully small, and our knowledge of the concentrations and dosage schedules that might be effective are so incomplete that I cannot foresee much success for the clinical studies currently going on. This is unfortunate since the interferon is definitely an effective and nontoxic inhibitor of cell growth in many systems that have been studied. Such a remarkable substance needs more careful study than the rapid buildup and almost certain letdown that cancer chemotherapy with interferon seems to be receiving. At present, my one hope here is that the large commercial investment that has been expended to clone human interferon genes will dictate that strong efforts be made to find some use for all the interferon to be produced. In this case, for once economics may dictate for the good of medicine and science.

Certainly, negative preliminary results should not dishearten clinical oncologists from pushing on with studies of interferon. When more interferon is available, studies using varied dose schedules should be employed on a number of different types of tumors. It would certainly be important to find out whether treatment with human interferons might be effective on Burkitt lymphomas, nasopharyngeal carcinomas, or hepatomas. The first two appear to be associated with infection by the Epstein–Barr virus, the last in some cases, with human hepatitis B virus. The possible virus association of these tumors makes them good candidates for trials with human interferons. Other types of tumors may also be sensitive to interferon treatment; however, it may be possible to develop *in vitro* tests for sensitivity to interferon treatment by growing tumor cells in culture and testing them under such conditions.

Interferon treatment will probably also be aggressively attempted in more virus diseases. I have already discussed the special reasons why arbovirus and rabies virus infections may be favorably affected by interferons. These diseases are not important medical problems in the areas of the world that can afford to undertake such clinical studies, but humanitarian considerations should prompt the initiation of such studies where they may be of great help in dealing with serious medical problems.

I have also mentioned that treatment with interferons might be attempted in some diseases in which a viral etiology is suspected. Multiple sclerosis and other slow degenerative diseases of the central nervous system are prime candidates for such efforts. In a way, such treatment would be not only therapeutic but also diagnostic. If the treatment were effective, this would be a strong argument in favor of a viral factor as a cause of the disease. Such studies will probably be forthcoming

As interferons become more available, the clinical finding of Merigan and Hirsch on the therapeutic uses of interferon in cancer patients and transplantation recipients can also be expected to find application. In addition, more studies employing interferon in other immunocompromised patients should be carried out. The suppression of *Herpes zoster* in cancer patients may decrease hospitalization time. Treatment of this disease with interferon in noncancer patients might also be attempted, as the pain associated with the disease is often severe and persistent and interferon treatment has been found to decrease postherpetic neuralgia. In the case of transplantation patients, interferon may serve several useful functions. It is thought by some that frequently infections with the herpes viruses, human cytomegalovirus, or the Epstein-Barr virus may contribute to the rejection of renal transplants. Such virus infections in transplant recipients can also be lethal in themselves. If interferon inhibits the growth of these viruses, it may contribute to the success of transplants. In addition, as mentioned earlier, the immunosuppressive activity of interferons may be helpful in preventing graft rejections, although this may be balanced by the ability of interferon to activate natural killer cells.

More studies on interferon's role in the pathogenesis of disease will certainly be undertaken. Gresser's work on the effect of interferons on the diseases associated with long-term lymphocytic choriomeningitis virus (LCMV) infection in mice suggests that in some cases interferons may have a role in inducing or exacerbating a disease state. Circulating interferon (probably gamma interferon) has also been discovered in patients with active diseases involving the immune system such as rheumatoid arthritis or disseminated lupus erythematosis (DLE). Might not the interferon produced contribute to the development of the joint disease or renal disease that play such an important part, respectively, in rheumatoid arthritis or DLE? If it is possible that the kidney disease in LCMV infections is related to the interferon production induced by the virus, is it not possible that gamma interferon induced by the abnormal immune reactions in DLE may be related to kidney damage in this disease?

Interferons may play important and hitherto unsuspected roles in other disease states and future research will elucidate some of these. As previously discussed, there is a finding which suggests that interferon production may be important in the development of asthma during the course of viral infection. Since interferons induce fever, it is possible that they also play a role in the development of the febrile response associated with virus diseases. Indeed, since bacterial products, certain bacteria (including the double-stranded RNA forms often present in fungi), and other microorganisms induce interferon production, it is possible that the fever seen in diseases with many infectious agents is, at least in part, mediated by the interferon they induce. Therefore, interferons may be found to play a role in the pathogenesis of several disease states.

Next to be considered here are the roles of interferons in cell biology. This area has expanded so rapidly that it must be approached with caution. There will probably be attempts to find relationships between the variously described effects of interferons. For instance, we know that interferons modify cell growth and differentiation processes. We also know that interferon treatment induces intracellular enzymes. Are these enzyme activities related to the effects of interferons on cell growth and differentiation? Are cell growth and differentiation at all related to the changes induced in membranes by interferon treatment? It seems possible that all of these may depend on one another. Interferon may bring about alterations in the plasma membrane; these changes may in turn lead to induction or inhibition of key enzyme systems, which in turn could have important effects on cells. There is wide scope for research in these areas.

In a way Ian Kerr has turned this problem inside out. Some of his current findings suggest that the synthetase and kinase induced by interferon treatment are important in several systems. For instance, when estrogen is withdrawn from hen oviduct tissue, a rapid fall in protein synthesis ensues; this fall correlates well with a rise in the level of 2',5'-A synthetase. Thus, the findings in the interferon system may have wide application in such diverse fields as endocrinology and hematology, where kinases and synthetases identical to those induced by interferon treatment are present in differentiating red cells. Thus, studies with the effects of interferons may have increased our insights in diverse physiological systems and will probably continue to do so.

The mention of the field of endocrinology reminds one of how many similarities there are between the actions of interferons and of polypeptide hormones. These will certainly be further explored. Although interferons are not produced by special endocrine organs, as are conventional hormones, the binding and early steps in development of antiviral activity appear to resemble those of polypeptide hormones. If indeed cyclic AMP and prostaglandins have a role in the development of interferon action, this would be one more similarity between interferons and hormones. Finally, the development of the effects of interferon appears related to the induction and inhibition of specific intracellular enzymatic activities. In this respect, too, the activities of interferons are reminiscent of those of hormones.

The genetics of the production of interferons should interest many scientists. The work of the De Maeyers has provided a basis for the concept of multiple gene control for interferon production in mice. Early results in the cloning of human and mouse alpha and beta interferon genes suggest the existence of multiple copies of genes for each of these types of interferons. Perhaps the different subgroups of alpha and beta interferons have somewhat different functions. It is possible that the varying effects of interferon preparations may each be due to a specific interferon. This problem requires further elucidation and will undoubtedly receive it. Investigation of this finding may provide important insights into gene structure, organization, and function.

Interferons also seem to have a significant role as regulators of the immune system. One important question for present and future research is whether gamma interferons are produced as specific immunoregulators that possess antiviral activity as a secondary function. It will be interesting to find out whether the induction of polyadenylate synthetase or the protein kinase contributes to interferon's role in the immune response. It is also possible that the effects on the immune system are secondary to interferon's activity on cell membranes. In addition, if interferon does have a significant antitumor activity, future research will have to determine how much of this activity is due to the regulatory effect of interferons on the immune system.

Finally, something should be mentioned about the original effect described for interferons, their antiviral activity. Understanding of interferon's production and role as a natural antiviral agent has progressed to the point where one can predict that future progress in this area of research will be useful in helping us to understand some aspects of cell biology and resistance to virus diseases. Our studies on the mechanism of action of interferons, however, have provided too many mechanisms of interferon action. The answer to the problem posed by the plethora of antiviral activities may be that they are all operative, but in an infection of a cell with a specific virus, this does not preclude the possibility that one particular mechansim may be of prime significance. It would then, of course, be incorrect for an investigator to claim that this is the sole mechanism of interferon's antiviral activity.

It seems, therefore, that progress in the understanding of antiviral activities of interferons will depend on the recognition that interferons induce many different antiviral activities. If a virus can escape from one or more of these, perhaps an additional activity may still inhibit an important phase of the virus replication cycle, and, therefore, inhibit virus growth. Future work in this area must define which mechanism of action is important in specific viral infections.

SUMMARY

1. Interferons are assayed on the basis of the antiviral state that they induce. Such assays are extremely sensitive because of the very great biological activity of interferons—less than one-trillionth of a gram of interferon can be detected. Unfortunately, like most biological assays, they are less accurate and reproducible than are chemical assays.

2. Production of interferons is induced by viruses or by a number of nonviral substances. The production of interferons is tightly controlled by cells, so that its study has resulted in insight into animal cell biology. Human cells produce three forms of interferon.

3. The antiviral state induced by interferons is complex. Interferon treatment results in the induction of cellular enzymes that act to inhibit the production of virus proteins. This results in decreased virus growth. In addition, interferon treatment inhibits assembly of some viruses. This results in the production of noninfectious virus particles that cannot then go on to infect new cells. Thus, virus growth is limited by both mechanisms.

4. Interferons also have several biological activities other than their ability to induce an antiviral state. They exercise control over the cells involved in the immune response. This effect may provide some new insights into this process and permit its modification in cases where this is desirable, such as in organ transplantation. Interferons also act as negative cell growth control factors. This property has prompted the experimental use of interferon as therapy for cancers.

5. Interferons appear to be natural antiviral substances that are at least partially responsible for recovery from some primary virus infections. Interferons are produced rapidly in response to virus infections. A deficiency in interferon production results in some cases in abnormally severe virus infections in experimental animals.

6. Because of the very small amounts of interferons that are produced by animal cells, very little has been available so far for clinical studies. What studies have been carried out, however, show promise. Interferons have been effectively employed to treat virus-induced acute respiratory infections, chronic liver infections by hepatitis B virus, and herpetic infections. In addition, there is preliminary evidence that the growth of some forms of human cancer may be slowed by treatment with interferon.

10
THE FUTURE IS NOW

The future has arrived for interferons, and we are presently involved in a reassessment of our thinking because of the large amount of pertinent information very recently gathered. This information has come through the application to interferon studies of two extremely powerful technologies that are revolutionizing almost all fields of biology—the cloning of animal genes in microorganisms and the production of monoclonal antibodies.

The cloning of genes for human alpha and beta interferons was carried out for the most part to produce more interferons for clinical studies. It could not have been anticipated how much our ideas about the organization of human genes in general and the genes responsible for interferon production in particular would be altered.

The cloning of human interferon genes has so far been carried out in the bacterium *E. coli*, but it will be of great interest to investigate whether other microorganisms can produce human interferons, or whether the genes for human interferons are active in the cells of other animal species. At any rate, *E. coli* produce both alpha and beta interferons after their genes have been integrated into the episomal DNA of the microorganism. The interferon produced collects in the periplasmic space between the bacterial cell wall and the cell membrane; thus, human interferons are not actually transported out of the bacterial cell. This makes for extremely rapid concentration, since the bacterial cells have only to be collected in order to obtain all of the interferon produced by the culture. The bacteria must then be lysed in order to release the interferon. This procedure does have the disadvantage of producing a "dirty" interferon preparation, one contaminated with many bacterial structural elements. With the recent progress in the purification of interferons, however, this has not proven to be an extremely difficult problem to solve; thus, quite purified preparations of interferons have already been obtained from bacteria.

Of course, the primary purpose for the cloning of human interferon genes was to obtain large amounts of human interferons for clinical and biological studies. So far it has been possible to obtain 0.1–0.5 mg of interferons per liter of bacterial culture. This means that much higher yields of human interferons are already possible under the presently existing cloning technology than could be obtained with production in human leukocyte or fibroblast cultures. With progress in optimizing interferon production by microorganisms, it is not unreasonable to predict that the problem of the short supply of interferons for clinical use will be solved in the near future.

One important issue has, however, already been resolved. The interferons produced by *E. coli* are biologically active. The human alpha interferon made in *E. coli* has been shown to protect monkeys against EMC virus infection. Other interferons produced in *E. coli* have the characteristic activities of interferons on the immune system and on cell growth.

The promise of an increased supply of human interferons, one sufficient to permit the necessary clinical studies to prove or disprove the usefulness of human interferons in the therapy of various diseases, would more than justify the efforts and the expense that have gone into the cloning of human interferon genes. As an added bonus, however, the cloning procedure has given us insight into what appears to be a fascinating aspect of biology. Because the bacteria in which the interferon is produced must also replicate a DNA, which is complementary to interferon messenger RNA (cDNA) as they multiply, an almost infinite supply of interferon cDNA is now available. This can be easily sequenced so that it is possible to infer the amino acid sequences of the interferons coded for by the cDNA. It is also possible to employ the cDNA to locate sites on human chromosomes which carry the genetic information for human interferon production. The early results of such studies have been, to say the least, surprising.

The alpha and beta interferons turn out to be a group of related proteins. However, we do not yet have enough information about the gamma interferon to say much about its relationship to the other (alpha and beta) antigenic species. The alpha and beta interferons are not related antigenically, but there is about a 30% identity in the sequence of amino acids present in them. This probably means that the genes for alpha and beta interferons diverged from one another many millions of years ago and have over this time become quite dissimilar. There are, however, some segments that are preserved, and it can be inferred that these amino acid sequences contain important functional loci that must remain quite unaltered in order that the interferon retain its biological functions.

The amino acid sequences that have been obtained from analysis of the cDNAs for interferons agree with those that have been determined by chemical analysis of interferon preparations purified by the latest techniques of protein separation. Such chemical analysis indicated that there were several distinct subspecies of alpha interferons. Indeed, alpha interferons appear to be a group of closely related proteins with different genetic loci. So far at least eight to ten different alpha interferons have been identified; they differ by about 15% in their amino acid sequence. In addition, there are preliminary reports that there are at least two subspecies of beta interferons.

The interferon genes that have been studied have one unusual property in common. Most genes that have been subjected to analysis have some regions that are transcribed into messenger RNA, but are then eliminated from the messenger RNA before it is finally translated. The elimination is by excision of RNA sequences and subsequent splicing, much as an editor would do to finish a film or a tape for final production. These unexpressed regions of a gene, called introns, are therefore silent as far as the protein product coded for by the gene is concerned. Their function is unknown, but they seem to be present in the genetic loci of most proteins. The interesting fact about the alpha interferon gene loci is that they contain no introns, thus making them members (at present) of a select group of proteins. When more is understood of the nature and function of introns, it will be possible to understand why the gene loci for alpha interferons lack them.

One other important question that arises from the studies on the genetic structure of the interferon loci is why there are so many of them? Each of the interferons so far studied has the wide range of biological activity that has been reported for interferons as a group—they are all antiviral, they inhibit cell growth, and they regulate the immune system. The significance of the multiplicity of alpha interferons cannot, therefore, be that each interferon has a specialized function, e.g., one being antiviral and another anticellular; however, the different alpha interferons do have varying activities on cells of different species. For instance, some are active only on human cells; others have very significant activities on bovine cells. Most of the alpha interferons are inactive on mouse cells; one species, however, is equally active on mouse and human cells. It may be that such varied species activity reflects a variation in the target cells for the interferons, so that the different species of human alpha interferons may acquire some specificity by manifesting their activity in different types of tissues.

With the discovery of the different types of interferons and the ability to manipulate their production, it has been possible to produce hybrid types of alpha interferons that do not exist in nature. These artificial hybrids combine portions of the genome of one interferon with those of another to produce a protein that may have a unique combination of properties. This is truly genetic engineering in the real sense of the word. It will probably take a great deal of time to sort out the various combinations of the many types of interferons that are known. Perhaps interferons with even more biological activity than the natural products are possible. It may be that interferons with high tissue specificity will be developed; these may have therapeutic application if, for instance, they inhibit the growth of specific tumors. In short, anything is now possible with interferons, so that we must expect the unexpected.

Several seemingly irreconcilable disagreements may have been resolved by the developments in our recently acquired understanding of interferons. There has been some controversy, for instance, about the location of the gene for human beta interferon production. Several different chromosomes have been implicated, the best evidence being that the active locus is on human chromosome 9, as reported in Chapter 4; however, if there were indeed several loci for the production of human beta interferons, the varying reports of the locus would be explained. Each group might have been studying the production of a different type of beta interferon.

Also, the heterogeneity often observed in the chemical and physical properties of human alpha interferons can be explained. It is surely due to true molecular differences, not to variations in glycosylation. Indeed, human alpha interferons have little or possibly no carbohydrate. The role of the extensive glycosylation of beta interferons is not known. The beta interferon produced by *E. coli* is completely unglycosylated, but appears to have normal biological activity. If the carbohydrate should nevertheless be important, it can be added to the interferon produced by microorganisms by incubating such beta interferon preparations with cell-free extracts prepared from dog pancreas, a particularly rich source of glycosylating enzymes.

The availability of monoclonal antibodies to interferons has not yet had as spectacular an impact on the interferon field as have the results of cloning; nevertheless, significant advances have been made. Monoclonal antibodies to mixtures of human alpha interferons and to their various subspecies have been employed to purify interferons. In one preliminary study, a 5000-fold purification of alpha interferon was achieved in a single step using an antibody affinity column. It must be anticipated that the general availability of monoclonal antibodies to interferons will lead to their rapid and cheap purification, thus contributing to the potential clinical use of interferons.

Rapid assays for interferons employing monoclonal antibodies are also being developed. This would be real progress, because it will permit research on interferons to be carried out by clinical and basic science laboratories not set up for tissue culture studies. As pointed out previously, it may not be possible for immunoassays employing antibodies to interferons to approach the exquisite sensitivity of the biological assays now in use, but simplicity and rapidity must count for something; also, it is certainly not always important to employ the most sensitive assay available.

Finally, it is not unlikely that monoclonal antibodies to interferons will be employed for analysis of the functions of different regions of interferon molecules. It might be possible to determine active sites for binding and biological function through the use of monoclonal antibodies.

All in all, the period since I started this book has been a most exciting time in this field, and I do not anticipate that the pace of progress will slow down in the forseeable future.

GLOSSARY

Actinomycin D   An antibiotic that inhibits RNA synthesis dependent on a DNA template.

Adenosine triphosphate (ATP)   A high-energy phosphate that serves as the principal energy storage and transfer compound of the cell.

Allergy   A hypersensitive state acquired through exposure to a specific allergen.

Amino acids   The building blocks of proteins: there are 20 common amino acids.

Amino acid sequence   The order of the amino acids in a peptide or protein.

Antibody   A protein molecule produced in the body by lymphoid cells, particularly plasma cells, in response to stimulation by an antigen.

Antigen   A substance that elicits a specific immune response when introduced into the tissues of the body.

Arbovirus   A virus transmitted by insect bite (arthropod-borne viruses). Group A arboviruses are positive-stranded RNA viruses.

Assay   A method of quantitation for a substance such as an interferon.

Asthma   A chronic immune-related disease in which labored breathing and wheezing result from bronchospasm and excessive bronchial secretions.

Attenuated virus vaccine   A vaccine composed of living infectious virus that is of low virulence. Such organisms stimulate active protective immunity; however, they are incapable of producing serious disease.

Bone marrow   Soft connective tissues located in the cavities of the bones.

Bone marrow-derived cell (B cell)   A lymphoid cell that originated in the bone marrow, escaped the influence of the thymus, and is present in a lymphoid organ.

C-type particle   An RNA tumor virus defined on the basis of its appearance in the electron microscope. Viruses of this type are responsible for many sarcomas and leukemias in animals and chronic infections tn tissue cultures.

Cell culture   The *in vitro* growth of cells isolated from multicellular organisms.

Cell cycle   The sequence of events occurring in a cell in the period between mitotic divisions.

Cell-free extract   A fluid containing most of the soluble molecules of a cell, made by breaking open cells.

Cell-mediated immunity   Specific immunity that is mediated by small lymphocytes and is dependent on the presence of a thymus at birth.

Chromatography   Separatory procedure that exploits varying affinities of molecules for a substance.

Chromosomes   Intranuclear structures in which the hereditary material of cells and viruses is contained.

Clone   A family of cells descended from a single cellular ancestor and, therefore, genetically identical.

Coat protein(s)   The external structural protein(s) of a virus.

Codon   A sequence of three adjacent nucleotides that code for an amino acid.

Complementary   With reference to nucleic acids, base-paired.

Covalent bonds   Chemical bonds formed by the sharing of electrons between atoms.

Cyclic AMP   Adenosine monophosphate with phosphate group bonded internally (phosphodiester bond between 3' and 5' carbon atoms) to form cyclic molecule. Active in regulation of gene expression.

Cycloheximide   An inhibitor of protein biosynthesis that acts to slow up the elongation of peptide chains.

Cytopathic effect (CPE)   Virus-induced cell damage.

Cytotoxic antibody   An antibody that reacts with antigens present on a cell surface, which damages that cell or its surface.

Defective interfering particles (DIPs)   Noninfectious virus forms with truncated nucleic acids genomes. They may interfere with the growth of normal virus particles.

Delayed hypersensitivity   A cell-mediated immune reaction that normally reaches its peak about 24 hr after challenge.

DNA (deoxyribonucleic acid)   A polymer of deoxyribonucleotides. The genetic material of all cells.

Double-stranded RNA   An RNA form with two complementary strands of RNA.

Early and late proteins   Viral-specific proteins which are synthesized at characteristic times after infection.

Electron microscopy   A technique for visualizing material that uses beams of electrons instead of light rays. It permits greater magnification than is possible with an optical microscope.

Electrophoresis   A separatory procedure that exploits the varying migration of molecules in an electric field.

Encephalitis   An inflammatory disease of the brain.

Encephalomycarditis virus (EMC virus)   A mouse picornavirus related to poliovirus. It consists of a protein capsid containing a positive single-stranded RNA. The RNA freed from the capsid is infectious. Mengovirus is closely related to EMC virus.

Endogenous virus   A virus that exists in a proviral, partially inactive form within a host cell.

Endonuclease   An enzyme that makes internal cuts in DNA or RNA backbone chains.

Enzymes   A protein molecule capable of catalyzing a chemical reaction.

Fibroblasts   A differentiated cell that grows very well in culture and has the spindle shape and growth rate of connective tissue cells.

Freeze-fracture   To fracture frozen samples and then encase complementary surfaces in metal to view in the electron microscope.

Ganglioside   A glycolipid that is most often found on the outer surface of the cell membrane.

Gene   A stretch along a chromosome that codes for a functional product such as either RNA or its translation product, a polypeptide.

Genetic information   The information contained in a sequence of nucleotide bases in a DNA (or RNA) molecule.

Genome   A haploid set of chromosomes, with their associated genes.

Globulin   A class of proteins characterized by being insoluble in water but soluble in saline solutions.

Glomerulonephritis   An autoimmune disease in which the major damage is to the glomeruli of the kidney.

Glycolipid   A lipid containing a carbohydrate moiety.

Glycoprotein   A protein to which sugar residues are attached.

Golgi cisternae   A complex series of flattened, parallel membranes that function in molecular processing. Secretory products are packaged into vacuoles here.

Graft rejection   A cell-mediated immune reaction elicited by the grafting of genetically dissimilar tissue onto a recipient. The reaction leads to destruction and ultimate rejection of the transplanted tissue.

Graft-versus-host   A disease that results upon transfer of lymphocytes from an individual who is genetically dissimilar to the recipient.

Granulocyte   A leukocyte that possesses distinct cytoplasmic granules such as eosinophils, basophils, and neutrophils.

Growth curve   The change in the number of cells or viruses in a growing culture as a function of time.

Guanosine triphosphate (GTP)   A high-energy phosphate analogue of ATP. GTP is required for the initiation of protein synthesis.

Haploid state   The chromosome state in which each chromosome is present only once.

Hemagglutination   The property of causing red blood cells to attach to a surface.

Histocompatibility antigen   A genetically determined cell surface antigen.

HLA histocompatibility antigens   The cell surface histocompatibility antigens on human cells that are important in tissue transplantation and that are controlled by a single gene complex.

Host cell   A cell whose metabolism is used for virus growth and reproduction.

Humoral antibody   An antibody present in the blood serum and tissue fluid of the body.

Humoral immunity   Immunity mediated by specific antibodies present in the blood serum and tissue fluids of the body.

Hybridization of nucleic acid   The reannealing of single-stranded nucleic acid chains. The formation of double-stranded regions indicates complementarity of sequence.

Hydrolysis   The breaking of a molecule into two or more smaller molecules by the addition of a water molecule.

Hydrophobic   The property (possessed by certain molecules or functional groups) of being only poorly soluble in water.

Hypersensitivity   The state, existing in a previously immunized individual, in which tissue damage results from the immune reaction to a further dose of antigen. If tissue damage is severe, the condition may be referred to as one form of allergy.

IgE   An immunoglobulin normally present at very low levels in man but elevated in allergic diseases and in certain infections.

Immune response   The body's response to a foreign substance.

Immunoglobulin   Any globulin protein that is comprised of light and heavy chains. All antibodies are immunoglobulins.

Inducible substance   A substance, usually a protein, whose rate of production can be increased by the presence of inducers in the cell. Interferon production is an induced process.

Infectious viral nucleic acid   A purified viral nucleic acid that can infect a host cell and cause the production of progeny viral particles.

Initiation factor   A specific protein required for the initiation of protein synthesis.

Insertion   Addition of new bases between pre-existing bases on a nucleic acid chain.

Interference   The ability of one virus to interfere with the growth of another virus.

Interferons Proteins that exert a wide spectrum of antiviral activity in animal cells and also possess several biological activities other than the ability to induce an antiviral state. An interferon is often active only in cells of the animal species producing that interferon; cellular metabolic processes involving RNA and protein synthesis are required for interferon activity. Three types of interferons are described in this monograph; alpha, beta, and gamma (see Table IV).

In vitro Pertaining to experiments done in a cell-free system, also including the growth of cells from multicellular organisms under cell culture conditions.

In vitro protein synthesis The incorporation of amino acids into polypeptide chains in a cell-free system.

In vivo Pertaining to experiments carried out in animals.

Isoelectric focusing A separatory technique that depends on the varying charge on different molecules.

Leucocyte Any of the white cells of the blood.

Leukemia A form of cancer characterized by extensive proliferation of immature white blood cells (leukocytes).

Leukopenia A significant decrease in the level of circulating leukocytes.

Lymph nodes Small, pea-sized organs distributed widely throughout the body and composed mostly of lymphoid cells.

Lymphoblastoid cell A transformed lymphocyte that multiplies in an unregulated manner.

Lymphocyte A cell associated with all aspects of specific immunity. Lymphocytes are the chief constituents of lymphoid tissue.

Lymphoid tissue A body tissue in which the predominant cell type belongs to the lymphoid series, such as the spleen, lymph nodes, thymus, tonsils, adenoids, and circulating lymphocytes.

Lymphokine A factor released by antigenically stimulated T lymphocytes.

Lymphoma Cancer of lymphatic tissue.

Lysis The bursting of a cell by the destruction of its plasma membrane.

Lytic infection Viral infection leading to lysis of cell and release of progeny virus.

Lytic virus A virus whose multiplication leads to lysis of the host cell.

Macrophage Any of the diverse group of cells (except granulocytes) that have the capacity to engulf and destroy foreign material.

Memory cells A lymphoid cell that, because of an earlier encounter with an antigen, retains an increased reactivity to that antigen.

Messenger RNA (mRNA) RNA that serves as a template for protein synthesis.

Mitogen A substance capable of inducing DNA synthesis and division in lymphocytes.

Molecular weight The sum of the atomic weights of the constituent atoms in a molecule.

Monolayer A layer of cells that is uniformly one cell thick.

Monomer The basic subunit from which, by repetition of a single reaction, polymers are made.

Neuraminidase A viral enzyme that attacks a cell surface carbohydrate.

Nonspecific immunity Bodily defense mechanisms that do not specifically recognize antigens or mount specific immune responses, but that provide for the destruction and removal of foreign substances. Interferons are examples of nonspecific immunity.

Nucleases Enzymes that cleave nucleic acid chains.

Nucleic acid A nucleotide polymer.

2′,5′ oligoadenylates Polymers of adenosine synthesized from ATP by an enzyme, oligoadenylate synthetase. They have a 2′,5′-phosphate linkage with the general structure $pppA2'p5'(A)_m2'p5'A_{OH}$, where m is 1 or more. The adenosine trimer is the most common molecule present in tissues, but polymers up to hexamers and heptamers are present, all of which inhibit cell protein synthesis by activating an endonuclease that hydrolyzes RNA.

Oligoadenylate synthetase An enzyme which forms 2′,5′-oligoadenylate polymers from ATP.

Oocyte An unfertilized egg cell.

Peptide bond A covalent bond between two amino acids in which the amino group of one amino acid is bonded to the carboxyl group of the other with the elimination of H_2O.

Phagocyte A scavenger cell.

Phospholipids Lipids that contain charged, phosphate head groups. These are one of the primary components of cell membranes.

Picornavirus A small RNA-containing positive-stranded virus with a protein capsid and no membrane. Members of this group include EMC virus, mengovirus, and poliovirus.

Plaque A round clear area in a confluent cell sheet that results from the killing or lysis of contiguous cells by several cycles of virus growth. Interferon assays may be based on a reduction in the number or size of plaques caused by a given number of virus particles.

Plasma cell The predominant immunoglobulin-producing cell type of the lymphoid cell series.

Plasma membrane A membrane that encloses the cytoplasm; such membranes are semipermeable and composed of lipid and protein.

Polymerase An enzyme capable of catalyzing the polymerization of nucleic acids.

Polypeptide A chemical that yields amino acids when decomposed but that is smaller than a protein.

Polyribosome A complex of a messenger RNA molecule and ribosomes, actively engaged in polypeptide synthesis.

Primary response The weak response of the immunological system upon its first exposure to a given antigen.

Primary structure The number of polypeptide or nucleotide chains in a protein or nucleic acid, their sequence, and the location of inter- and intrachain bridges.

Prostaglandin One of a group of fatty acids capable of stimulating the adenylate cyclase system to produce cyclic AMP.

Protein A complex chemical substance made up of amino acids; proteins are essential constituents of all living cells.

Protein kinase An enzyme that adds phosphate groups to proteins.

Protein phosphatase   An enzyme that removes phosphate groups from proteins.

Provirus   The state of a virus in which it is integrated into a host cell chromosome and thus may be transmitted from one cell generation to another.

Radioimmunoassay   An immunologic procedure for measuring the concentration of antigen or antibody by employing radioactively labeled materials.

Receptor   A chemical structure on the surface of cells that binds and interacts with specific substances or viruses.

Regulatory gene   A gene whose primary function is to control the rate of synthesis of the products of other genes.

Repressible substance   A substance whose rate of production is decreased when the intracellular concentration of certain factors increases.

Repressor   A regulatory gene product, capable of combining with an inducer.

Reverse transcriptase   An enzyme coded by certain RNA viruses that is able to make complementary single-stranded DNA chains from RNA templates and then to convert these DNA chains to double-helical form.

Ribonuclease   An enzyme that can cleave RNA.

Ribosomal RNA (rRNA)   The nucleic acid component of ribosomes.

Ribosomes   Small cellular particles made up of rRNA and protein. Ribosomes are the site of protein synthesis.

Rickettsiae   Small, disease-causing, bacteria-like organisms that are obligate intracellular parasites. They contain DNA and RNA, as well as protein-synthesizing machinery.

RNA (ribonucleic acid)   A polymer of ribonucleotides.

RNA polymerase   An enzyme that catalyzes the formation of RNA from ribonucieoside triphosphates, using DNA as a template.

Rough endoplasmic reticulum   Extensive inner membranous sacs (endoplasmic reticulum) which have bound ribosomes. Secretory proteins are synthesized on these membrane-bound ribosomes.

Secondary response   The vigorous response of the immunological system upon exposure to an antigen previously encountered.

Serum (pl. sera) The liquid part of the blood remaining after cells and fibrin have been removed.

Serum protein Protein found in serum (cell-free) component of blood. Includes immunoglobulins, albumin, clotting factors, and enzymes.

Smooth endoplasmic reticulum Extensive inner membranous sacs (endoplasmic reticulum) that are free of ribosomes. They are a major site for attachment of sugar residues to nascent proteins to form glycoproteins.

Synthetic polyribonucleotides RNA made *in vitro* without a nucleic acid template, either by enzymatic or by chemical synthesis.

T antigen An antigen found in nuclei of cells infected or transformed by certain tumor viruses, usually SV40.

Temperature-sensitive mutation A mutation yielding a protein that is functional at low temperature, but is inactivated by temperature elevation.

Template The macromolecular mold for the synthesis of another macromolecule.

Thrombocytopenia A significant decrease in the circulating level of platelets.

Thymus A central lymphoid organ of major importance in the development of immune capability.

Thymus-derived lymphocyte (T lymphocyte) A small lymphocyte that attains new immunologic capabilities on (or after) residence in the thymus.

Transcription A process involving base pairing, whereby the genetic information contained in DNA is used to form a complementary sequence of bases in an RNA chain.

Transfer RNA (tRNA) Any of at least twenty structurally similar species of RNA each of which is able to combine covalently with a specific amino acid and to hydrogen-bond with at least one mRNA nucleotide triplet.

Transferases Enzymes that catalyze the exchange of functional groups.

Transformation The genetic modification induced by the incorporation into a cell of DNA viruses or provirus forms of RNA viruses.

Translation The process whereby the genetic information present in an mRNA molecule directs the order of the specific amino acids during protein synthesis.

Translational control Regulation of gene expression by controlling the rate at which a specific mRNA molecule is translated. Interferons appear to exercise translational control over virus-directed protein synthesis.

Trypsin A proteolytic enzyme, secreted by the pancreas, that cleaves peptide chains.

Tumor A mass formed by the uncontrolled proliferation of cells.

Tumor virus A virus that induces the formation of a tumor.

Vesicular stomatitis virus (VSV) A single, negative-stranded RNA virus of the rhabdovirus group.

Viral-specific enzyme A viral-specified enzyme produced in the host cell after viral infection. Some virus-specific enzymes are incorporated into the virus.

Virus An infectious disease-causing agent, smaller than a bacterium, which requires intact host cells for replication, and which contains either DNA or RNA as its genetic component.

Vital dye uptake The entry of certain dyes into living cells. This can form the basis for an assay of cell killing by a virus.

INDEX

U

V

X

Y